first place
4 health

Bible Study Series

better
together

Lucinda Secrest McDowell

Published by Gospel Light
Ventura, California, U.S.A.
www.gospellight.com
Printed in the U.S.A.

Caution: The information contained in this book is intended to be solely for
informational and educational purposes. It is assumed that the First Place 4 Health
participant will consult a medical or health professional before beginning this or
any other weight-loss or physical fitness program.

Library of Congress Cataloging-in-Publication Data
McDowell, Lucinda Secrest, 1953-
Better together / Lucinda Secrest McDowell.
p. cm. — (First place 4 health Bible study series)
ISBN 978-0-8307-5892-0 (trade paper)
1. Communities—Biblical teaching—Textbooks. 2. Christian life—
Biblical teaching—Textbooks. I. Title.
BS680.P43M34 2011
241'.67—dc22
2011005679

Rights for publishing this book outside the U.S.A. or in non-English
languages are administered by Gospel Light Worldwide, an international
not-for-profit ministry. For additional information, please visit
www.glww.org, email info@glww.org, or write to Gospel Light Worldwide,
1957 Eastman Avenue, Ventura, CA 93003, U.S.A.

To order copies of this book and other Gospel Light products in bulk
quantities, please contact us at 1-800-446-7735.

contents

BIBLE STUDIES

ADDITIONAL MATERIALS

about the author

Lucinda Secrest McDowell, a graduate of Gordon-Conwell Theological Seminary, is an international conference speaker and author of 10 books, including the First Place 4 Health Bible Studies *God's Purpose for You* and *Fit and Healthy Summer*. Her other books include *30 Ways to Embrace Life, Spa for the Soul, Amazed by Grace* and *Role of a Lifetime*. She has also written for 50 magazines and been a contributing author to 25 other books. A wife and mother of four, Cindy writes and speaks from New England through her ministry "Encouraging Words that Transform." She leads a First Place 4 Health class for women and men in the Hartford area and is also part of a First Place 4 Health authors group, helping to coordinate their annual wellness week. Visit her website www.EncouragingWords.net or contact her at cindy@encouragingwords.net.

foreword

My introduction to Bible study came when I joined First Place in March 1981. I had been attending church since I was a small child, but the extent of my study of the Bible had been reading my Sunday School quarterly on Saturday night. On Sunday morning, I would listen to my Sunday School teacher as she taught God's Word to me. During the worship service, I would listen to our pastor as he taught God's Word to me. Frankly, the idea of digging out the truths of the Bible for myself had never entered my mind.

Perhaps you are right where I was back in 1981. If so, you are in for a blessing you never dreamed possible. As you start studying the truths of the Bible for yourself through the First Place 4 Health Bible studies, you will see God begin to open your understanding of His Word.

Almost every First Place 4 Health member I have talked with about the program says, "The weight loss is wonderful, but the most important thing I have received from my association with First Place 4 Health is learning to study God's Word." The First Place 4 Health Bible studies are designed to be done on a daily basis. As you work through each day's study (which will take 15 to 20 minutes to complete), you will be discovering the deep truths of God's Word. A part of each week's study will also include a Bible memory verse for the week.

There are many in-depth Bible studies on the market. The First Place 4 Health Bible studies are not designed for the purpose of in-depth study, but are designed to be used in conjunction with the rest of the program to bring balance into your life. Our desire is for each member to begin having a personal quiet time with God each day. This time alone with God should include a time of prayer, Bible reading and Bible study. Having a quiet time is a daily discipline that will bring the rich rewards of balance, which is something we all need.

God bless you as you begin this exciting journey toward a balanced life. God will richly bless your efforts to give Him first place in your life. Remember Matthew 6:33: "But seek first his kingdom and his righteousness, and all these things will be given to you as well."

Carole Lewis, First Place 4 Health National Director

introduction

First Place 4 Health is a Christ-centered health program that emphasizes balance in the physical, mental, emotional and spiritual areas of life. The First Place 4 Health program is meant to be a daily process. As we learn to keep Christ first in our lives, we will find that He is the One who satisfies our hunger and our every need.

This Bible study is designed to be used in conjunction with the First Place 4 Health program but can be beneficial for anyone interested in obtaining a balanced lifestyle. The Bible study has been created in a five-day format, with the last two days reserved for reflection on the material studied. Keep in mind that the ultimate goal of studying the Bible is not only for knowledge but also for application and a changed life. Don't feel anxious if you can't seem to find the *correct* answer. Many times, the Word will speak differently to different people, depending on where they are in their walk with God and the season of life they are experiencing. Be prepared to discuss with your fellow First Place 4 Health members what you learned that week through your study.

There are some additional components included with this study that will be helpful as you pursue the goal of giving Christ first place in every area of your life:

- **Group Prayer Request Form:** This form is at the end of each week's study. You can use this to record any special requests that might be given in class.

- **Leader Discussion Guide:** This discussion guide is provided to help the First Place 4 Health leader guide a group through this Bible study. It includes ideas for facilitating a First Place 4 Health class discussion for each week of the Bible study.

- **Two Weeks of Menu Plans with Recipes:** There are 14 days of meals, and all are interchangeable. Each day totals 1,400 to 1,500 calories and includes snacks. Instructions are given for those who need more calories. An accompanying grocery list includes items needed for each week of meals.

- **First Place 4 Health Member Survey:** Fill this out and bring it to your first meeting. This information will help your leader know your interests and talents.

- **Personal Weight and Measurement Record:** Use this form to keep a record of your weight loss. Record any loss or gain on the chart after the weigh-in at each week's meeting.

- **Weekly Prayer Partner Forms:** Fill out this form before class and place it into a basket during the class meeting. After class, you will draw out a prayer request form, and this will be your prayer partner for the week. Try to call or email the person sometime before the next class meeting to encourage that person.

- **Live It Trackers:** Your Live It Tracker is to be completed at home and turned in to your leader at your weekly First Place 4 Health meeting. The Tracker is designed to help you practice mindfulness and stay accountable with regard to your eating and exercise habits. Step-by-step instructions for how to use the Live It Tracker are provided in the *Member's Guide*.

- **Let's Count Our Miles!** A worthy goal we encourage is for you to complete 100 miles of exercise during your 12 weeks in First Place 4 Health. There are many activities listed on pages 255-256 that count toward your goal of 100 miles. When you complete a mile of activity, mark off the box listed on the Hundred Mile Club chart located on the inside of the back cover.

- **Scripture Memory Cards:** These cards have been designed so you can use them while exercising. It is suggested that you punch a hole in the upper left corner and place the cards on a ring. You may want to take the cards in the car or to work so you can practice each week's Scripture memory verse throughout the day.

- **Scripture Memory CD:** All 10 Scripture memory verses have been put to music at an exercise tempo in the CD at the back of this study. Use this CD when exercising or even when you are just driving in your car. The words of Scripture are often easier to memorize when accompanied by music.

welcome to
Better Together

At your first group meeting for this session of First Place 4 Health, you will meet your fellow members, get an overview of your materials and find out what you can expect at weekly meetings. The majority of your class time will be spent learning about the four-sided person concept, the Live It Food Plan, and how change begins from the inside out. You will also have a chance to ask any questions about how to get the most out of First Place 4 Health. If possible, complete the Member Survey on page 205 before your first group meeting. The information that you give will help your leader tailor the next 12 weeks to the needs of the whole group.

Each weekly meeting begins with a weigh-in for members. This will allow you to track your progress over the 12-week session. Your Week One weigh-in/measurement will establish a baseline of comparison so that you can set healthy goals for this session. If you are apprehensive about weighing in every week, talk with your group leader about your concerns. He or she will have some options for you to consider that will make the weigh-in activity encouraging rather than stressful.

The day after your first meeting, begin Week Two of this Bible study. This session, you will look at 10 "one anothers" found in the Bible and discover the truth of how to live in community through loving, serving, encouraging, forgiving and honoring one another—developing all the godly characteristics necessary to become better together! As you open yourself to the truth of Scripture and share your hopes and struggles with the members of your group during the next 12 weeks, you'll find yourself becoming the healthy child of God you are designed to be!

better together in love

SCRIPTURE MEMORY VERSE
And this is his command: to believe in the name of his Son, Jesus Christ, and to love one another as he commanded us.
1 JOHN 3:23

Those of us in First Place 4 Health know that it is in community that we learn to live healthy lives focused on balancing the physical, spiritual, mental and emotional areas of life. We cannot do this alone—although many of us have tried. In *Better Together* we will be exploring the many "one anothers" found in God's Word—those times when believers are exhorted to behave in such a way that both honors God and those around us—our community.

The apostle Paul used the Greek word *allelon* (translated "for one another") more than 40 times in his letters to instruct the believers in the Early Church on their mutual responsibilities toward fellow Christ followers. Of the 10 specific "one anothers" that we will be studying this session, the first and most important is this week's command to "love one another." Love was the only "one another" Jesus specifically commanded, and He considered it so important that He referred to it in at least 15 different verses.

If you think that you know all there is about loving others, well, perhaps this week you will be pleasantly surprised to discover a new way to reach out in love to those around you.

Day
1

OBEDIENT

Dear heavenly Father, thank You for putting all of Your commands—such as love one another—in Your Word. Please help me to obey You in all I do and say. Amen.

According to 1 John 3:23, our memory verse this week, what are two of God's commands?

1. *To Believe in the name of Jesus*
2. *To Love One Another*

According to John 14:15,21, what two things cannot be separated?

1. *Loving God*
2. *Obedience*

Read Deuteronomy 7:12. What will the result be of obeying and doing what God commands?

The Lord will keep His covenant of love with us.

Read Leviticus 26:3-13. What are some of the specific blessings that God promises for obedience to Him?

Rain for the crops - fruit in the trees, "Food" abundance - Harvest - Safety in the Land - Peace, No fear, Safety - no animal attacks. Destruction of Enemies - many babies, His presence among us. Freedom - Liberty!

Jesus also described a benefit of obedience. What is this benefit, and how does Jesus emphasize the importance of it (see John 15:10)?

We will remain in His love

According to Romans 13:8, how do we know we have fulfilled God's law of obedience?

If we love one another.

In seeking balanced health in the physical, spiritual, mental and emotional areas of life, most of us already know—at least in general—what *to* do and what *not* to do. In what area of life do you struggle most to obey? Why is that area particularly difficult for you?

Exercise - Unable to do it w/ others - need to be taught how + have accountability - Don't like to do it alone.

*God, please forgive me for the times I have been disobedient
and gone my own way. Help me to follow Your way of truth and love.
I want to obey You in all areas of my life. Amen.*

HEARTFELT · Day 2

*Almighty God, You created me to have a heart that
cares for others, even though it might sometimes be broken.
May I use my heart to love deeply in Your power. Amen.*

Yesterday we discovered that loving one another is a command of God—one that calls for our full obedience. Peter actually points out in 1 Peter 1:22-23 that our obedience is an act of purification. What does he say to do next?

Love one another - by Gods power through His Word!

In today's culture, the word "love" is used in every context from "I love pizza" to "I love my children." When expressed for such a wide variety of things, the meaning becomes watered down and loses its punch. Read 1 Corinthians 13:1-3. What happens if we do not love "deeply from the heart"?

Our actions mean nothing. Our works - even use of our gifts mean nothing. They are empty & lifeless, even our sacrifice means nothing. It must come from the heart.

According to 1 John 3:14, what is the worst that happens if we don't sincerely love others?

We remain in death & have no life. No eternal life. We know that we have passed from death unto life when we can genuinely love one another. Love is the greatest - main ingredient of the Christian life.

Can you think of a time when you tried to act in love toward someone, but your heart really wasn't in it? Describe the results.

Ann Skains

Resentment replaced love - wanted to get away & have nothing to do w/ that person to avoid being hurt - division - loss of a friend. Feeling alone & uncared for.

Read 1 Peter 4:8. Think of a time when you continued to love someone even though it was really hard to do. How did your experience flesh out the words of this verse?

Michael my husband

He responded eventually with amazement & realized he wanted me in his life - he needed me.

Is there someone you are loving only superficially right now—someone whom God wants you to love from the heart? If so, begin to pray for that person daily. That's a great way to start loving in a heartfelt way.

God, all too often I love only as much as it is convenient for me to do. Help me go the extra mile and be more sincere and intentional with others. Amen.

EXEMPLARY Day 3

*Father God, You have loved me so much that You gave Your only
Son to die for my sins. I cannot comprehend such love, but I ask that
You begin to help me love others in a similar sacrificial way. Amen.*

According to 1 John 3:16, what is the ultimate expression of sincere love?

_____

_____

_____

Why did Christ urge His disciples to love one another (see John 13:34-35)?

_____

_____

_____

In later years, as the Church was growing, Paul urged the new community to follow Christ's example of love. Read Romans 5:8-10. How did God show His love for us through His Son, Jesus Christ?

_____

_____

_____

This act of death and resurrection was an example of true love in action, What is one way that you can "die daily" to your own will and your own way in order to show love for someone else? Give one practical example.

_____

_____

_____

Every time we allow ourselves to be inconvenienced in order to help others, we are laying down our lives—our time, our own needs and our wills—and are saying that the other people are more important than we are.

When we model Jesus' behavior, we are not merely servants, or agents, following orders. Instead, what does Jesus call us (see John 15:14-15)?

_____

_____

_____

Why is this better than being a servant?

_____

_____

_____

Dear Lord, You know that deep down I can be selfish. Please show me opportunities to "lay down my life" for others today. Amen.

Day 4 — ENDURING

God, I get so discouraged because so much around me seems changeable, fickle and not reliable. Thank You for being the One who will be here forever. Amen.

Perhaps the most amazing characteristic of biblical love (and the one in stark contrast to our culture's view of love) is that love endures. True love is not a fickle, ever-changing commodity that we offer and then retract on a whim. Instead, God calls us to a love that sticks it out over the long haul.

First Corinthians 13 is the apostle Paul's great treatise on love. As you read through verses 1-13, write down all the characteristics mentioned in verses 4-8 (yes, there are 16!)

1. Love is _____
2. Love is _____
3. Love does not _____
4. Love does not _____
5. Love is not _____
6. Love is not _____
7. Love is not _____

   8. Love is not _____

   9. Love keeps _____

 10. Love does not _____

 11. Love _____

 12. Love always _____

 13. Love always _____

 14. Love always _____

 15. Love always _____

 16. Love never _____

Read 1 Corinthians 13:8. What are three things that do come to an end?

  1. _____

  2. _____

  3. _____

Have you ever been in a love relationship that did *not* endure? Why do you think that love did not last?

_____

_____

_____

Read Psalms 6:4; 86:5. How is God's love different from the human love we both give and receive?

_____

_____

_____

What do you need to do to make your love more like God's?

_____

_____

_____

> *God, I confess that I have given up on love too many times. May I trust You*
> *to empower me to love others in a persevering way—a love that never fails.*

Day 5

FAMILIAL

Father, I am so glad that I am part of Your forever family. Help me to be loving to all around me, even if I don't always know how to begin. Amen.

According to Romans 12:10, how should we love others?

_____

_____

_____

Here Paul introduces a powerful new metaphor for our love—a familial one. The original Greek term Paul used is *philadelphia* ("brotherly love"), which commonly referred to family relationships. Beginning with the book of Acts, the New Testament writers used a portion of this word, *adelpho*, approximately 220 times to refer to the church family. Literally translated as "from the womb," this term emphasizes the importance of being related to one another by being "born again" into God's eternal family. Read Hebrews 13:1. According to the author of Hebrews, how should members of the Church family treat each other?

_____

_____

_____

Most people who have brothers and/or sisters did not always get along while growing up. Given this, why do you think we are told to love each other "as brothers"?

_____

_____

_____

What examples of the command in Hebrews 13:1 are given in verses 2-3?

_____

_____

_____

Which do you think is harder: acting lovingly toward strangers, prisoners and the mistreated, or acting lovingly toward your own family? Why?

_____

_____

_____

_____

Look up 1 Thessalonians 4:9-10 and fill in what Paul states about how the believers were to love one another.

> Now about _____ _____ we do not need to write to you, for you yourselves have been taught by God to _____ _____ _____.
> And in fact, you do _____ _____ ____ _____ throughout Macedonia. Yet we urge you, brothers, to do so more and more.

How does your *Better Together* Bible study group function as a family?

_____

_____

_____

_____

Father, I am Your child and I need Your guidance and wisdom in order to live out Your family values. Thank You for showing me the way. Amen.

REFLECTION AND APPLICATION

Day
6

Loving God, I realize that loving others is a huge task and not always easy. Relationships are fraught with miscommunications and misunderstandings. Help me to understand more and more so I may love more and more. Amen.

As we seek to love one another, let's keep in mind that each of us communicates love in a different way. Dr. Gary Chapman describes the primary way we communicate love to another person (and the way we want to receive love) as our love language:

1. Words of affirmation. Some people prefer to express their love—and have love expressed to them—through verbal compliments and affirming statements.

2. Quality time. Some people find and give love through undivided attention. When they are with someone they love, they are completely with them—in mind, body and spirit.

3. Receiving gifts. Some people express and receive love through presents. . . . The gifts don't necessarily have to be expensive. What they want is a visual symbol of love, something they can hold in their hands, evidence that their spouse was thinking of them.

4. Acts of service. Some people communicate their love by doing things to make life easier for their spouse. By the same token, they prefer to have love expressed to them in the same way.

5. Physical touch. Some people prefer to express love and have love expressed to them through physical contact, whether it's kissing, caressing, hugging, holding hands, or high-fiving.[1]

While this exercise was originally designed to help married couples, it can help you identify where you are on the spectrum with others. For instance, if your love language is words of affirmation and another's is acts of service, you will be on opposite ends of the spectrum. You may not feel the person loves you because he or she is not speaking words of affirmation to you, while that person may not feel you love him or her because you are not doing acts of service. The problem is in the way each of you expresses love.

Which of the five love languages do you most embrace? Why?

_____

_____

_____

_____

What do you think is the love language of each person with whom you live and with whom you spend the most time?

_____

_____

_____

How can you determine whether another person speaks a love language different from your own? How can knowing that person's love language help you in your relationship?

_____

_____

_____

How can we love one another if we don't take time to understand other people and to listen and know them better? This is truly one of the great keys to loving others. As you understand their fears and joys, you will discover numerous ways to reach out in love.

Jesus, I need to be intentional about knowing others and helping them to know me too. Thank You for giving me courage to pursue this path. Amen.

REFLECTION AND APPLICATION

Day 7

Dear God, I do want to live in a more balanced way so that I have more energy and more to give others. Thank You for being with me on my journey. Most of all, thank You for staying with me all the way. Amen.

Congratulations! You are near the end of the first week of *Better Together* and are well on your way to a healthier lifestyle that honors God and those in your community. Throughout this study, you will be stretched in learning how to reach out and be there for those around you. In the process, not only will you bless them, but also you will be blessed.

If you're going through *Better Together* in a First Place 4 Health group, perhaps one of the best features of your class is the large group sharing time. It's great to learn what works for others as far as healthy snacks, eating out, exercise options and so forth. Success stories—and, yes, even failure stories—are ways people lead by example when they share their experiences with others. What have you heard from someone else in your group lately that was of particular help to you?

_____

_____

_____

_____

How did this represent a blessing or an act of love in your life?

_____

_____

_____

_____

Dr. Catherine Hart Weber says that we flourish, grow and become our most authentic and best self in the presence of God's love and the company of one another. In other words, we truly are better together!

> From birth, healthy attachments are crucial for development—our brain, emotions, body and relationships. We are hardwired for being in meaningful relationships, and when we are not, we don't flourish as God intends. Focus on building healthy relationships. Listen to others. Interact in a way that involves mutual sharing of experiences, thoughts, feelings, hopes, and dreams. Learn healthy ways of relating, even arguing. Discover your and others' styles of attachment, of relating, love languages, and other factors that will help you improve your ability to cultivate meaningful healthy relationship attachments. Resolve and repair disputes and conflict. Be willing to take responsibility for your failings, let go of grudges, and forgive.[2]

How do you expect to develop your love in the four areas of your life?

Physical

_____

_____

_____

_____

Spiritual

_____

_____

_____

_____

Emotional

_____

_____

_____

_____

Mental

_____

_____

_____

_____

Lord, Your love for me is so great that You sacrificed Your Son for me. Help me to obey You and love others with a sincerity that reflects Jesus' example of unfailing love. I want Your love to be seen as I love other people. Amen.

Notes

1. Gary Chapman with Randy Southern, *The World's Easiest Guide to Family Relationships,* World's Easiest Guides (Chicago: Northfield Publishing, 2001), pp. 43-44.
2. Catherine Hart Weber, *Flourish: Discover the Daily Joy of Abundant, Vibrant Living* (Minneapolis, MN: Bethany House Publishers, 2010), p. 44.

Group Prayer Requests

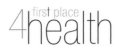

Today's Date: _____

Name	Request

Results

_____
_____
_____
_____
_____
_____

better together in service

Last week we learned that Jesus Christ is our model for loving one another. This week we discover the same thing is true for serving one another—we serve one another because Christ humbled Himself to become a servant to us. Service is often hard work and often goes unrecognized and unrewarded, but it is something we do to show God's love to others, not for any sort of personal gain.

Did you know that the basic concept of service is used over 300 times in the New Testament? What a contrast to our modern me-first society— most people today feel that they are entitled to be served, not that they should serve others. For those of us who want to begin to serve others in an intentional way, sometimes we don't know where to begin.

Mother Teresa, who served the dying in Calcutta through the Missionaries of Charity, offers some insight in this area: "I never look at the masses as my responsibility. I look only at the individual. I can love only one person at a time. I can feed only one person at a time. . . . I picked up one person. . . . The whole work is only a drop in the ocean. But if we don't put the drop in, the ocean would be one drop less. Same thing for you. Same thing in your family. Same thing in the church where you go. Just begin. One. One. One."[1]

GRACE

Heavenly Father, help me to faithfully administer the grace You have given me so that others will be served. Amen.

Read Ephesians 2:8-9. Because grace is an undeserved gift from God (not a reward that is earned), what should be our attitude about offering grace to others?

In the Old Testament, "grace" was translated from a Hebrew word that means to stoop. Theologian Donald Barnhouse said that "love that goes upwards is worship; love that goes outward is affection; love that stoops is grace."[2] Has God ever offered His grace by stooping down to lift you up? If so, briefly describe such a time.

What does 1 Peter 4:10, our memory verse, say about how we can administer God's grace to others?

There are many spiritual gifts listed in the Scriptures. Below is a list of gifts as described in Romans 12, 1 Corinthians 12 and Ephesians 4. Circle the gifts that you believe God has given you.

administration	evangelism	giving
apostle	exhortation	healing
discernment	faith	helps

knowledge   pastor   tongues
leadership   prophecy   tongues interpretation
mercy   service   wisdom
miracles   teaching

How are you using your gifts to serve others?

_____

_____

_____

_____

According to Colossians 1:5-6, what evidence is there that people have understood God's grace?

_____

_____

_____

_____

How might your extending grace to others influence their belief in God?

_____

_____

_____

_____

If grace is an undeserved gift from God (not a reward that is earned), then how should that affect our attitude about offering grace to others?

_____

_____

_____

_____

Martin Luther King Jr. once said, "Anybody can serve. You do not have to have a college degree to serve. You do not have to make your subject and verb agree to serve. You only need a heart full of grace, a soul generated by love."[3]

> *Lord, thank You for the grace You have given to me and keep giving to me each time I ask for Your forgiveness. Help me to use my gifts to extend grace to others so that You are glorified. Fill my heart with grace that spills over. Amen.*

Day 2 HUMILITY

Christ, You humbled Yourself in order to serve me. Help me to be willing to live in humility so that others' concerns are more important than mine. Amen.

Throughout the Bible, God points out that humility is a fitting characteristic for His followers to possess. The Latin root of "humility" is *humus,* meaning from the earth. It can be a great compliment to say that someone is "down to earth." It means the person is approachable and not too lofty. This is the kind of humility that is necessary to serve one another. What does Peter say all disciples of Jesus should do (see 1 Peter 5:5)?

_____

_____

_____

Look up each verse and write down what God does for the humble.

Scripture	What God does for the humble
Psalm 18:27	
Psalm 25:9	
Psalm 147:6	
Psalm 149:4	
Proverbs 3:34	
Luke 1:52	
Luke 14:11	

Read Philippians 2:3-4. How does a humble person feel about others, and how is this attitude displayed in his or her life?

_____

_____

_____

How does this kind of action differ from the "selfish ambition" and "vain conceit" mentioned in verse 3?

_____

_____

_____

Thank You, Jesus, for Your life, which is a tangible reminder of putting others first. Help me to develop a willing and humble spirit as well. Amen.

AVAILABLE · Day 3

Father, help me to take the time to be aware of the needs around me. Help me to take the time to be available and to fill those needs in practical ways.

We cannot serve others unless we are available to them. Due to modern technology, most of us are available in numerous ways—cell phone, email, Facebook and, of course, in person. Okay, so at least we can be contacted. But when contacted by someone else with a need (assuming they were brave enough to ask us) are we truly available to follow through?

In John 12:26, Christ teaches us how to "be there" for others. Read John 12:26 and write down His statements.

Whoever serves Christ must _____

Christ's servant will be _____

The one who serves Christ will be _____

One Greek word used frequently in the New Testament to refer to serving others is *diakoneo*. *Diakoneo* means to minister to someone by caring for his or her material needs, but it can be expanded to caring for any area of need. This is where we get the word "deacon." In what ways do deacons serve in a church setting? How can we serve as deacons to one another?

_____

_____

_____

Read the story found in Mark 2:1-5,10-12. How did some friends make themselves available to help someone in need? What did they do?

_____

_____

_____

What did their friend most need at this time?

_____

_____

_____

When one way was blocked, what creative strategy did these friends use in order to serve their friend's needs? What was the result?

_____

_____

_____

An important part of the First Place 4 Health program is using the weekly prayer partner forms (see back of this book). When you have received this form, have you made yourself available and taken the time to pray through the request every day? Is there anything else you can do—any other way that you can make yourself available—to help in the situation?

_____

_____

_____

How can you be available this week and help someone you know who has a need?

_____

_____

_____

Father, who do you want me to "carry" to Jesus this week? Please open my heart so that when I know about a need, I make myself available to fulfill it.

LABOR   Day 4

Lord, labor as a way to serve others is a blessing for me and for those I serve. Please guide me to forget myself and remember Your Son's example. Amen.

To serve another requires that we expend time, energy and resources on behalf of someone in need. It also means that we labor in a spirit of honoring the other person above ourselves. This was demonstrated at a Promise Keepers pastors' conference in Atlanta a few years ago. Bishop Wellington Boone was preaching to the 40,000 pastors when he suddenly stopped and turned to fellow pastor Tony Evans, who was on the platform with him. "Tony," he said, "I'm willing to wash your feet in order to serve you."

In a matter of minutes, something spontaneous happened. Several men in the audience placed a makeshift container on the platform and filled it with a few bottles of water. They gave Wellington Boone a piece of cloth—probably some kind of T-shirt. He knelt before Tony Evans, removed his shoes and socks, and began washing his feet—all the time telling this brother in Christ that he loved him and wanted to serve him as a fellow pastor.[4] This was a true mark of humility and captured what Jesus had in mind when he told his disciples to serve one another.

Read John 13:1-17. What did Jesus do?

_____

_____

_____

In the culture of Jesus' time, everyone wore sandals and consequently had dirty feet. Thus it was the lowliest servant of each household whose job it was to wash the feet of each guest. This was not considered a privilege but a menial and lowly, yet necessary, task. Given this, why do you think Peter was vehement in not wanting Jesus to wash his feet?

_____

_____

_____

Washing the feet of the disciples was one of Jesus' final labors of love. What five takeaway messages was He trying to get across to them (see verses 15-17)?

1. I've set _____

2. You should _____

3. No servant is _____

4. No messenger is _____

5. If you do these things, you _____

Organizations that build homes and schools for others are always in need of volunteers. Have you ever helped do such labor? What did you do and how did it make you feel?

_____

_____

_____

Not all of us are physically able to do actual labor, but in what other ways could a person of limited means or abilities help with labor?

_____

_____

_____

Jesus, it's hard sometimes to labor as a way to serve others. Help me to willingly and cheerfully follow Your example, even when I think it's hard. Amen.

SELFLESS

Dear God, sometimes I let what I think I need overwhelm me, and I neglect the needs of those around me. Show me the way to serve others. Amen.

To serve one another, we must focus beyond our own self and our own needs. We must become selfless. Some have chosen to use the acronym **JOY** to illustrate the principle of selflessness: **J**esus first, **O**thers next, and **Y**ourself last. What acronym would aptly reflect your current behavior?

_____

_____

_____

One Greek word used in the New Testament to define selfless servants is *douleo,* which means to be a slave and to submit. This can also mean serving God and others in Christian love. But *douleo* can also mean being enslaved to something else. This word is used 160 times in the New Testament to illustrate someone who has given himself to another's will. What does Paul say about this in Romans 6:6?

_____

_____

_____

Paul uses the same word in Galatians 5:13. What command does he give at the end of the verse?

_____

_____

_____

Earlier in this verse, Paul issues both a statement and a warning. What are they?

_____

_____

_____

How can similar cautions be applied to your efforts to pursue a healthy and balanced lifestyle?

_____

_____

_____

_____

Lord, please help me not to focus on my own needs but on the needs of others. Thank You that I can trust in You to meet my needs. Amen.

Day
6

REFLECTION AND APPLICATION

Gentle Savior, You are the One who gathers us up in Your arms of love and care. May my response be to live my life as a testimony of Your love by doing Your work and serving others each day. Amen.

Teresa of Avila, a sixteenth-century nun, once wrote, "Christ has no body now on earth but yours; yours are the only hands with which He can do His work. Yours are the only feet with which He can go about the world; yours are the only eyes through which His compassion can shine forth upon a troubled world. Christ has no body on earth but yours."[5] If we are indeed to be the hands, feet, eyes and body of Christ in today's world, we must be intentional about serving others. Think again about the gifts, the talents, God has given to you that we first looked at in Day One. How can you expand the use of these gifts to extend God's grace to others?

_____

_____

_____

_____

Catherine Weber tells a story about an evening when she was rushing to pick up dinner for her family on her way home, and she picked up the very last rotisserie chicken at the store. On the way to the car, she saw a man rummaging in the trash and was filled with compassion. When she offered to buy him something to eat, to her dismay all he wanted was one of those cooked chickens:

> It was all just too bizarre. He had to choose the thing that would cost me the most.
>
> It took me a few seconds to process my thoughts. "I don't want to be a bother," he said. It was then that I realized I needed to just give him the chicken. "I would be glad to give you a chicken. In fact, I have one here in my car. Let me get it for you. . . ."
>
> Each day we face the challenge of listening to the voice of the Spirit of God leading us to give up our time, our expectations, our selfish ways and our stuff. Jesus modeled this for us. He was always in tune with the voice of the Father—to the extent of giving up His life for us.[6]

If you had been in Catherine Weber's situation, would you have given away your family's dinner? Would you even have approached the man? Why or why not?

_____

_____

_____

_____

When have you been stretched to show kindness and compassion by serving someone? What did it cost you?

_____

_____

_____

_____

> *Lord, please help to make me a person with a servant's spirit. Help me to be the kind of person who willingly and cheerfully gives to others. Amen.*

REFLECTION AND APPLICATION

Savior, You have sent people to touch my life in numerous ways. Help me to move beyond my own concerns to a place where I can truly serve others. Amen.

This week, we have looked at five different aspects of what serving one another involves. As you review each one today, write next to it something specific you can begin to do, through God's power, that would show this aspect of service.

Grace

_____

_____

_____

Humility

_____

_____

_____

Availability

_____

_____

_____

Labor

_____

_____

_____

Selflessness

_____

_____

_____

As you conclude this week's session, take a moment to pray this prayer from Richard Foster about being willing to serve others regardless of the cost.

God, today I resonate with the desperate cry in the Gospel, "I believe, help my unbelief." Sometimes I think I operate my life out of more doubt than faith. And yet I want to believe . . . and I do believe.

Increase faith within me, O Lord. I'm sure that for faith to grow You will put me in situations where I'll need resources beyond myself. I submit to this process.

Will this mean moving out on behalf of others, praying for them and trusting You to work in them? If so, then show me the who, what, when, and where, and I will seek to act at Your bidding. Throughout I am trusting You to take me from faith to faith—from the faith I do have to the faith that I am in the process of receiving.

Thank You for hearing my prayer. Amen.[6]

Notes

1. Mother Teresa, quoted in Peter Scazzero, *Daily Office* (Elmhurst, NY: Emotionally Healthy Spirituality, 2008), p. 122.
2. Donald Barnhouse, quoted in Walter A. Boyd, "Christian Conduct in a Modern World," *Assembly Testimony Magazine,* March/April 2002. *http://www.assemblytestimony.org/?q=node/35* (accessed April 12, 2011).
3. Martin Luther King, quoted in Marcia Ford, "Essentials for Life," (Nashville, TN: Thomas Nelson Publishers, 2010), p. 95.
4. Gene Getz, *"Building Up One Another,"* (Colorado Springs, CO: David C. Cook Publishers, 1997), p. 42.
5. Teresa of Avila, quoted in Thomas Becknell and Mary Ellen Ashcroft, eds., *The Pursuit of Wisdom: 125 Prayers from Timeless Voices* (Valley Forge, PA: Judson Press, 2002) p. 150.
6. Catherine Hart Weber, *Flourish: Discover the Daily Joy of Abundant, Vibrant Living* (Minneapolis, MN: Bethany House Publishers, 2010), p. 113.
7. Thomas Becknell and Mary Ellen Ashcroft, editors, *The Pursuit of Wisdom* (Valley Forge, PA: Judson Press, 2002) p. 91.

Group Prayer Requests

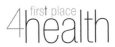

Today's Date: _____

Name	Request

Results

_____

_____

_____

_____

_____

_____

better together in patience

SCRIPTURE MEMORY VERSE

Be completely humble and gentle; be patient, bearing with one another in love.
EPHESIANS 4:2

Patience is hard to practice, but it is something God commanded us to have because He knows we are better off when we are patient people.

Now that we are on Week 4 in our *Better Together* study, have you begun to see positive changes from your making healthier lifestyle choices, or are you discouraged that results aren't coming quickly enough for you? It's easy to give in to impatience and want to bypass the process in order to reach our goals quickly. But that's not usually the path toward lasting change. We must learn to be patient with ourselves and with one another.

Impatience breeds stress, worry and a tendency to get shortchanged out of the positive benefits that come to those who wait. This week we are going to seek God's help to develop a spirit of patience—with ourselves and with others.

LONG-SUFFERING
Day 1

God, I don't want to "suffer long" for results—I want them now! I do realize, though, that most important achievements are hard fought and deliberate, so help me be patient. Amen.

Patience doesn't come naturally to most of us. But just as Christ deals patiently with us, He expects us to follow His example. According to

1 Timothy 1:16, what did Christ do for Paul?

_____

_____

_____

What was the outcome?

_____

_____

_____

_____

What four commands are found in 1 Thessalonians 5:14?

1. _____

2. _____

3. _____

4. _____

To whom is Paul speaking? To whom is he asking patience to be extended?

_____

_____

_____

_____

Why is the word "patience" often translated as "long-suffering"?

_____

_____

_____

When have you experienced long-suffering?

_____

_____

_____

_____

Read James 5:7-8. What example of patience is found in this passage?

_____
_____
_____
_____
_____

According to Ephesians 4:2, our memory verse, we are to display patience by "bearing with one another in love." Describe a few practical ways of "bearing with one another in love."

_____
_____
_____
_____
_____

Divine Father, please help me to recognize that change and growth is a process. Help me to submit to Your will and Your way so that in due time, as I practice patience, I may reap a harvest of righteousness. Amen.

AFFLICTION
Day 2

God, our comforter, You know how hard it is to be patient when I am troubled by pain or confusion or problems of one sort or another. Help me to wait and trust that You indeed are in control. Amen.

Perhaps it is hardest to be patient when we are in the middle of difficulties, pain or suffering of some sort. Why do you think this is so?

_____
_____
_____
_____

What are the three commands found in Romans 12:12?

1. _____
2. _____
3. _____

How can hope and prayer help us be more patient?

_____
_____
_____

King David shared a personal struggle about dealing with affliction in Psalm 40. When David was troubled, what was the first thing he did (see verse 1)?

_____
_____
_____

As a result, what three things did God do?

1. _____
2. _____
3. _____

Because of what God did, what will happen (see verses 3-4)?

_____
_____
_____

Paul also experienced his fair share of affliction. However, in Romans 5:3-5 Paul states that he rejoiced in his sufferings. What three things does Paul state are produced by suffering?

1. _____
2. _____
3. _____

If we, too, appropriate this kind of patience during the afflictions of our lives, what will be the result (see verse 5)?

_____

_____

_____

Author and speaker Carol Kent has written that during her times of affliction:

> The best [gifts] have come disguised in suffering I would never choose, and they are priceless: the comfort of a friend who cries with me when my heart is breaking, the joy of watching my son grow deep in his faith, the opportunities to encourage people who are hurting, and the privilege of connecting people to the real source of hope: the Rock I cling to—God Himself.[1]

What is your greatest affliction at this time? Even as you identify it, give it to the Lord in prayer and ask Him to grant you patience to endure it and wisdom to recognize that good can come from it.

Lord, help me recognize that sometimes the best gifts are disguised in afflictions I would never have chosen to suffer. Help me to use them for Your glory.

MEEKNESS   Day 3

Heavenly Father, most of the world doesn't value those who are meek. Help me to understand that being meek is a positive step toward patience. Amen.

What words come to mind when you hear "meek"?

_____

_____

_____

Write down the dictionary definition of "meek."

_____

_____

_____

_____

When Jesus said, "I am gentle and humble in heart," His words were translated from the same root word from which we get "meek" (Matthew 11:29). Choosing to follow Christ on this path is actually a sign of strength, not weakness, according to Bible teacher Jennifer Kennedy Dean:

> The meek put their full trust in the Lord and wait for His work in His way at His time. The meek do not trust in their own ability nor do they act in their own strength.
>
> The Lord knows that it often appears that the loud, brash and overbearing inherit the land. It sometimes looks like those who trust in themselves win the day. But it is not really so, He says. Pride has in it the seeds of its own destruction. The meek have the strength to wait it out and to let God work. The meek have learned that pride is weakness and meekness is strength.[2]

Read Matthew 5:5. Why would Jesus' words be considered somewhat radical?

_____

_____

_____

_____

What does God say He will do for the humble (the meek) in Psalm 25:9?

_____

_____

_____

One of the reasons it's so hard to be meek is that most people are not, yet they seem to be doing just fine. This is beautifully addressed in Psalm 37. What three commands are given in verse 7?

1. _____
2. _____
3. _____

What happens to us when we begin to fret about how everyone else seems better off (see verse 8)?

_____
_____
_____
_____

According to verses 9-11, what happens to these two kinds of people?

1. _____
2. _____

According to 1 Peter 3:4, what is of great worth in God's sight?

_____
_____
_____
_____

What is one thing you could do today in order to start being meek?

_____
_____
_____
_____

Father, help me work on my inner spirit so that its beauty shines through and brightens my whole demeanor. I want access to all the benefits You have for those who show strength through meekness. Amen.

Day 4

WISDOM

God of infinite wisdom, please make me wise so that I may discern how to wait patiently on Your timing for all good things. Amen.

What is the difference between knowledge and wisdom?

_____

_____

_____

Who is the wisest person you know still living today? What makes that person wise?

_____

_____

_____

Throughout the Bible—and actually throughout our daily lives—we see the results of impatience and foolishness. Conversely, those who exhibit patience to one another are considered wise. Read Proverbs 14:29. What are the characteristics of a patient person?

_____

_____

_____

Now read Proverbs 15:18. According to this passage, what are the characteristics of a quick-tempered person?

_____

_____

_____

Can you recall a time when you were quick-tempered? What happened?

_____

_____

_____

According to Proverbs 19:11, what is the source of patience, and what is the result?

_____

_____

_____

_____

_____

What does James 1:5 say about how we obtain godly wisdom?

_____

_____

_____

_____

Of course, we don't want to get so enthralled with our own wisdom that we become prideful. What did King Solomon, the wisest man who ever lived, say is better than pride (see Ecclesiastes 7:8)?

_____

_____

_____

_____

If you struggle with your temper, how can you learn to gain wisdom and be more patient?

_____

_____

_____

_____

_____

Lord, it's hard to keep praying for a result I have yet to see and experience. Please give me the wisdom I need to patiently wait for Your timing to work out Your perfect plan for me. Amen.

ENDURANCE

Dear Jesus, You who endured so much, help me to keep on keeping on, even when I feel like giving up. Remind me of the benefits of a balanced life. Amen.

Perhaps the greatest quality of patience is endurance. Throughout the New Testament, what we read as "endurance" is a translation of the Greek word *hypomone. Hypomone* means "a patient, steadfast waiting for" or "a patient sustaining or perseverance." Keep that in mind today as we look at what Paul had to say about patient and steadfast waiting.

Patience is needed when we don't have answers or results as quickly as we desire. Where have you needed more patience in your own First Place 4 Health endeavors recently?

_____

_____

_____

_____

Read Colossians 1:10-11. Where does Paul say our endurance and patience originate?

_____

_____

_____

_____

Patiently waiting for something is part of living "a life worthy of the Lord" (verse 10). What do you not yet have in your own life for which you must steadfastly wait on the Lord?

_____

_____

_____

_____

_____

Read 2 Corinthians 6:4-10. Paul listed many difficulties in his life, each of which provided an opportunity to depend on God and to endure with patience. Describe a few of the difficulties Paul had to patiently endure.

_____

_____

_____

_____

What opportunities for endurance do you have right now?

_____

_____

_____

_____

Even though Paul had to endure many hardships, what did he do when he felt "sorrowful" (verse 10)?

_____

_____

_____

_____

Even though Paul was poor, how did he make "many rich" (verse 10)?

_____

_____

_____

_____

Even though Paul had nothing, why did he believe he possessed "everything" (verse 10)?

_____

_____

_____

_____

Even though you may be steadfastly waiting for many things in your life, why should you, like Paul, believe you already possess "everything"?

Thank You, Father, for giving me strength to bear so much. Thank You for the apostle Paul who was an enduring witness who inspires me today. Amen.

Day 6 — REFLECTION AND APPLICATION

Father, You know that there are things I'm just itching to do or have happen right away. But even Your Son waited patiently until His time had come. May I only proceed with Your blessing and at Your pace. Amen.

Although we've talked quite a bit about Paul this week—what he had to say about patience and how he is a good example to follow in regard to patience—the primary model for our behavior is always Jesus. As Stephen W. Smith states in *Embracing Soul Care:*

> He waited about thirty years before He even began His revolutionary public ministry. From our North American perspective, we wonder what Jesus could have accomplished if he had started earlier and had longer to minister. But Jesus waited. He waited in the wilderness. He waited in the garden. He waited for His own execution. He waited in the tomb. Jesus learned the rhythm of waiting. We must learn the same rhythm if we are to grow, change, and become like Jesus. Although it seems inefficient, waiting is a necessary step toward spiritual maturity. Waiting cannot be bypassed, as much as we might wish that it could. We cannot become like Jesus overnight.[3]

We all strive for patience at times—with ourselves and with others. But if we follow Jesus' example, patiently waiting until the time is right for change to happen, we can bear with one another, endure affliction and humbly turn to God for help. How can Jesus' life help you be patient in your own life?

_____

_____

_____

_____

In his letter to the Colossians, Paul urged the believers to seek the truth and live as God wants them to, no matter what troubles arise:

> We pray that you'll have the strength to stick it out over the long haul —not the grim strength of gritting your teeth but the glory-strength God gives. It is strength that endures the unendurable and spills over into joy, thanking the Father who makes us strong enough to take part in everything bright and beautiful He has for us (Colossians 1:11-12, *THE MESSAGE*).

Why do you think that even though you might have a few setbacks, you will be able to reach your First Place 4 Health goals?

_____

_____

_____

_____

Where have you needed more patience in your own First Place 4 Health endeavors recently?

_____

_____

_____

_____

Ask God to be with you in the process and to help you learn lessons of His grace and patience all along the way.

Jesus, Help me to be an example of someone who waits patiently for change to happen. Help me learn how to bear with others who aren't moving as quickly as I would like so that they see Christ in me, the hope of glory. Amen.

Day
7

REFLECTION AND APPLICATION
Forgive me, Lord, for those times I do not give You my energy and resources. Help me to continually spend time to get to know You better. Amen.

Do you set aside time to be with God one day a week? God designed a rhythm to our lives—one that would help us stay balanced physically, spiritually, emotionally and mentally: We are to work and then rest. We are to engage and then disengage. We are to get involved and then with-draw. After all, what did God do when He had finished His work of creating the world and everything in it? In fact, God thought the Sabbath was important enough to include an instruction about it in the Ten Commandments. Read Exodus 20:8. Exactly what did God command?

_____
_____
_____

Why is this command so important (see Exodus 20:9-11)?

_____
_____
_____

What did Jesus have to say about the Sabbath (see Mark 2:27)?

_____
_____
_____

God designed the Sabbath as a time for us to go at a much slower pace than normal. Every other day we work and rush and accomplish much, but achieving and busyness are not applauded on the Sabbath. Stephen W. Smith, founder of The Potter's Inn Retreat Center, elaborates:

> This significant day encourages us to manage time in a different way. Because this particular day is kept, certain activities become rituals. We keep a commitment to family or community. Perhaps close friends come for dinner, or we visit them. We share being together. Meals during the week are more time conscious. A Sabbath meal can be a lingering experience of food and fellowship. We may spend time reading, napping, praying, talking—hatever slows us down and touches our soul.[4]

What would contribute to the Sabbath purpose of restoring your soul?

_____

_____

_____

_____

Dear God, I need Your help to be patient and wait on Your timing. Help me to rejoice when I must endure a hardship. Let me come humbly to You for Your help and guidance, seeking Your wisdom and will for my life. Help me to be patient with others and with myself. I want to depend on You more than on myself. Amen.

Notes
1. Carol Kent, *Between a Rock and a Grace Place: Divine Surprises in the Tight Spots of Life* (Grand Rapids, MI: Zondervan Publishers, 2010), p. 197.
2. Jennifer Kennedy Dean, *Set Apart: A Six-Week Study of the Beatitudes* (Birmingham, AL: New Hope Publishers, 2009).
3. Stephen W. Smith, *Embracing Soul Care: Making Space for What Matters Most* (Grand Rapids, MI: Kregel Publishers, 2006), p. 223.
4. Ibid., p. 139.

Group Prayer Requests

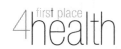

Today's Date: _____

Name	Request

Results

_____

_____

_____

_____

_____

Week Five

better together in fellowship

SCRIPTURE MEMORY VERSE
Let the word of Christ dwell in you richly as you teach and admonish one another with all wisdom, and as you sing psalms, hymns and spiritual songs with gratitude in your hearts to God.
COLOSSIANS 3:16

One of the best parts of being *better together* is the fellowship! Working through this study by gathering with others on a weekly basis to review the topics and examine practical goals for balanced health physically, spiritually, mentally and emotionally is itself a good step toward wellness.

And when everyone is gathered together, the fellowship can be contagious. We are reminded that we are not alone in our quest or in our struggles. We share ideas and challenge each other as "iron sharpens iron" (Proverbs 27:17). We "rejoice with those who rejoice; [and] mourn with those who mourn" (Romans 12:15). Mostly, we have each other's backs in prayer. Such aspects of fellowship are a biblical mandate and, as we will see this week, an essential ingredient in the life of faith.

Even though the Church was not launched officially until the Day of Pentecost, the ability of Christ followers to function in proper relationship with one another certainly began when Jesus was on earth. The disciples were first called "Christians" at Antioch (see Acts 11:26), a term that literally meant "belonging to Christ." Apparently, even nonbelievers recognized those who were Jesus' followers because their behavior reflected Jesus (see Acts 26:28).

We should ask ourselves if others can recognize us as followers of Christ because of our behavior—how we fellowship with one another and in the way we treat others.

Day 1 — OVERFLOW

Dear Lord, sometimes I have less-than-friendly feelings and responses to those around me. Please help me guard my heart so that what overflows from me is pleasing to You. Amen.

We fellowship with one another when our lives spill over into others' lives. According to Luke 6:45, what did Christ observe about a person's words and where they come from?

_____

_____

_____

_____

_____

What most often overflows from your heart to others?

_____

_____

_____

_____

_____

A wise person once said, "Garbage in, garbage out." According to Colossians 3:16, this week's memory verse, with what does Paul suggest we fill ourselves?

_____

_____

_____

_____

In what three ways are we encouraged to do that in this verse?

1. _____

2. _____

3. _____

Even as we choose to enjoy fellowship with others, we also enjoy fellowship with the trinity—God the Father, Jesus Christ His Son, and the Holy Spirit. According to 1 Corinthians 1:9, with whom has God called us into fellowship?

_____

_____

_____

_____

In 2 Corinthians 13:14, Paul says that the fellowship of the Holy Spirit will be with us. How do you best experience fellowship with God?

_____

_____

_____

_____

As you read 1 Corinthians 1:8-9, what does this warning bring to mind? Have you ever let anything "overflow" from you—anything you've said or done—that might have been detrimental to someone in your fellowship? If so, how can you prevent that from happening in the future?

_____

_____

_____

_____

Great God, may I always seek to be a unifier and not a divider among people. Help me to make fellowship a priority for Your sake, for the sake of others and for my own sake. Amen.

HOSPITALITY

*Thank You, God, for giving me a place to call home. May I never
take it for granted and may I always extend a welcome to others,
even as You welcome me into the home of Your heart. Amen.*

What is the difference between hospitality and entertaining?

_____

_____

_____

In Acts 5:42, we are told that the believers in Jerusalem met from "house
to house," as they had no permanent place to meet as a group. Pastor
Gene Getz elaborates:

> Their numbers increased so rapidly that no building was large
> enough to hold them. To complicate matters, the Jewish temple
> soon became "off limits" because of a serious theological rift be-
> tween the Jews who believed that Jesus Christ was the true Mes-
> siah and those who did not. This lack of permanent meeting
> facilities continued to be a problem for Christians in the New
> Testament culture for years.[1]

Despite this, why did the Early Church (as described in Acts 2:46-47)
continue to grow daily?

_____

_____

_____

_____

What does Paul command us to do in Romans 12:13?

_____

_____

_____

Read 1 Peter 4:9. How is hospitality to be offered?

_____

_____

_____

_____

Read Hebrews 13:2. Although the word "entertain" is used here, what reason is given for treating others in a generous and cordial manner?

_____

_____

_____

_____

Jesus taught that every time we reach out to others, we are ministering to Him as well. Read Matthew 25:35-36. In what ways can a person be hospitable by focusing on others?

_____

_____

_____

_____

Based on this passage from Matthew, in what new ways can you practice hospitality?

_____

_____

_____

_____

Do you ever suffer from CHAOS (Can't Have Anyone Over Syndrome)? Do you believe that before you can practice hospitality, your house must be spotless, you must learn to be a gourmet cook, your furniture must be reupholstered, you have to buy new dishes, and on and on and on?

Stop with the excuses and just reach out! How would your practice of hospitality change if you stopped focusing on yourself?

_____

_____

_____

Father, may I do away with pride and stop worrying about what others think of me and my home so that I can reach out in hospitality to anyone at any-time. Thank You that whatever I do for others, I also do for Jesus. Amen.

Day 3 — WORSHIP

King of Kings, truly You are worthy of my praise and thanksgiving and worship. I bow down to give You the honor and glory due Your name. Amen.

In Psalm 95:6-7, what are we encouraged to do and why?

_____

_____

_____

To worship, we must focus wholly on God and His character. The easiest way to do this is through praise, thanksgiving and adoration. The psalms are full of worshipful tributes to God, and that's probably why many Christ followers use psalms liberally in both personal devotions and corporate services. Look up each of these references and jot down the ways we are to praise and worship God.

Scripture	Ways to praise and worship God
Psalm 54:6	
Psalm 63:4	
Psalm 66:4	

Scripture	Ways to praise and worship God
Psalm 71:23	
Psalm 105:2	
Psalm 149:3	
Luke 14:11	

Which of these ways would be new for you? How can you incorporate this new way in how you worship?

_____

_____

_____

_____

Both the Hebrew and Greek words for "worship" mean to "prostrate one-self"—something rarely seen except in monasteries. The Hebrew word most frequently used in the Old Testament, *shachah*, can also mean "to bow down" or "to do reverence." The Greek word *proskuneo* also means "to kiss the hand." Regardless of how one chooses to worship, it is important to remember that it can take place anywhere and at any time. Robert Webber once said:

> A right ordering of God, the world, self, and neighbor is experienced, and the worshiper receives a peace that passes understanding. Simply put, worship is an it-is-well-with-my-soul experience.[2]

While daily worship of God is a good habit to start, why should we also worship with others (see Hebrews 10:25)?

_____

_____

_____

Lord of Lords, there are so many ways to show You worship. Forgive me
when I hold back and focus more on myself than on You. Help me to
encourage others to worship You as well. Amen.

Day 4 INSTRUCTION

Teacher, You have all wisdom and knowledge, yet You still equip us so we too
can impart wisdom to others. Thank You for using me this way. Amen.

One of the best benefits of life together in community is that we can
come alongside one another and urge one another on to greatness. This
is where gathering together for instruction and teaching becomes beneficial. Read Acts 5:42. What did members of the Early Church do daily?

_____

_____

_____

_____

_____

According to 2 Timothy 3:16-17, what is the ultimate source of instruction for godly living, and why is it so useful?

_____

_____

_____

_____

Which of God's instructions do you have the most trouble obeying? Why
does that one tend to be so difficult for you?

_____

_____

_____

_____

_____

In this day and age, there are many out there eager to instruct us—all the way down the wrong path! And often their teachings are couched in terms and references that sound okay. Obviously, you should not believe everything you hear. Read 1 John 4:1-2. What are we supposed to do with what we hear?

_____

_____

_____

_____

_____

What does Paul say in 1 Timothy 6:3-5 about people whose instructions are false and misleading?

_____

_____

_____

_____

Before you joined First Place 4 Health, did you ever start to follow someone's instructions about a quick way to achieve self-improvement only to later realize that the quick fix was quite false? How could being in close fellowship with other believers have helped you at that time?

_____

_____

_____

_____

_____

What is Paul convinced of about the church in Rome (see Romans 15:14)?

_____

_____

_____

_____

How has your involvement with First Place 4 Health improved your ability to instruct others?

_____

_____

_____

_____

_____

> *Help me, Lord, to be able to discern truth from falsehood so that*
> *I may always follow Your way and teach others with Your words*
> *and Your heart and in Your truth. Amen.*

Day 5 — COMMUNITY

Heavenly Father, I thank You that I do not journey alone but in community, a family of believers. Thank You for creating this community so that we can help each walk in the light. Amen.

In any community there are always posers—people who pretend to be committed in order to gain from the association. Read 1 John 1:5-7,9-10. How does John contrast the posers and the believers?

Posers	Believers

Paul witnessed the effects of people of darkness mixing in with people of light. What did Paul say believers should do in regard to unbelievers (see 2 Corinthians 6:14)?

_____

_____

_____

_____

Some people find this confusing because Christ taught us to reach out to unbelievers, but there is a difference between *knowing* unbelievers and being *yoked* together with them. What are some ways you can help each other in your community both to reach out but also to be careful about associations that drag you down?

_____

_____

_____

_____

The Early Church was a model of the kind of community Christ advocated. What attributes did those early believers have (see Acts 4:32)?

_____

_____

_____

_____

Community means communal, or having in common. In what ways can today's Church exhibit a community spirit similar to that of the Early Church?

_____

_____

_____

_____

Part of living in fellowship and in community involves thinking of others more than ourselves. What does Paul encourage the strong to do in Romans 15:1-2?

_____

_____

_____

How specifically can you carry out Paul's suggestion in the next few days?

_____

_____

_____

God, You know I sometimes struggle with ownership and possessions. Help me to be willing to offer them up to others in the spirit of fellowship. Amen.

Day 6 — REFLECTION AND APPLICATION

Mighty God, may I learn to worship You not only in my heart but also in community with others. May I serve others every single day of the week as an added act of worship. Amen.

As we learned earlier this week, an important aspect of fellowship is worshiping together. But is there a difference between worship service and the service of worship? Nashville area pastor Scotty Smith had this to say regarding the difference:

> As a kingdom of priests, we are expected to mature as God's worshipers in our service of worship, while celebrating the Lord Jesus' person and work through the ministry of the Word, the sacraments, prayer, praise, and fellowship. But we are also charged to incrementally restore God's broken worship by offering ourselves to God as "living sacrifices," as a people who accept the calling to the lifestyle of worship service, wherever God has placed us or will send us. . . . I'm now convinced that we've

placed an inordinate and unbiblical emphasis on our services of worship, largely to the exception of worship service.[3]

Whether or not you agree with Smith's observation, if worship is to focus on giving glory to God (whether in a service or through serving), how are you finding this balance in your own church and life?

Smith also notes, "The highest worship we can offer God in this life is to live, love, sing, pray, study, spend, invest, and sacrifice in ways that will call as much attention as possible to the glory and grace of Jesus Christ. Make much of Jesus . . . make much of Jesus as lead worshipers and as worship leaders."[4] How are you living out a life of worship through your fellowship with one another?

Jesus, You called me into fellowship with Yourself, and I must follow Your example and willingly reach out to others and bring them in to where there is life and health and strength. Give me courage, please. Amen.

REFLECTION AND APPLICATION

Day 7

God, sometimes I cling to darkness because it seems easier or safer, even when I know it is the path to death, not life. Help me to walk in Your light and bring light and life to all around me who still walk in dark places. Amen.

We must not only seek to live in fellowship with our closest companions on our life journey, but we are also called to widen our spheres of influence to the community beyond our comfort zones. When Christians isolate themselves from others, they are often perceived as being afraid to mingle with the rest of society or as setting themselves apart as being superior to everyone else. But that is not how we are meant to be.

> Those who love God are called to bring light to those who live in spiritual darkness. You cannot do that if you remain in the shadows, never letting the light of God shine through you to those who desperately need it. Your church friends may represent your comfort zone, but God did not call you to be comfortable; he called you to be obedient. And that means taking his love to those in your sphere of influence. . . .
>
> One of the primary ways, though, [God reveals Himself to people] is through his people, spreading his love to those who have no idea how to find it otherwise. Every time you interact with people who do not know God, you are part of God's purpose for his people.[5]

When you interact with people, do you remember that you are God's representative, that you should always model Jesus? Even when you say nothing, your behavior speaks for you. When have you made a conscious effort to react in fellowship to someone outside your home or church setting? What happened, and how did you feel about it?

_____

_____

_____

_____

How do you think the other person felt?

_____

_____

_____

_____

Jesus told His followers that they "are the salt of the earth" and thus season society by giving people a taste of the kingdom of God (Matthew 5:13). When salt is mixed with impurities, it loses some of its saltiness. How can you keep your unique "seasoning" but also spread it around to spice up your world?

_____

_____

_____

_____

Lord, You call us to bring light to those who live in spiritual darkness. Please let my fellowship today bless You and draw people to the light of Christ that You have placed within me. Help me to be your representative and model Jesus' example wherever I am today. Help me to reach out to others in fellowship and actively demonstrate the love that You have demonstrated to us. Amen.

Notes

1. Gene Getz, *Loving One Another* (Colorado Springs, CO: David C. Cook Publishers, 2002), p. 131.
2. Robert Webber, quoted in Marcia Ford, *Essentials for Life: Your Back-to-Basics Guide to What Matters Most* (Nashville, TN: Thomas Nelson Publishers, 2010), p. 105.
3. Steven Curtis Chapman and Scotty Smith, *Restoring Broken Things: What Happens When We Catch a Vision of the New World Jesus Is Creating* (Nashville, TN: Integrity Publishers, 2005), p. 153.
4. Ibid., p. 173.
5. Ford, *Essentials for Life,* p. 187.

Group Prayer Requests

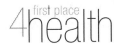

Today's Date: _____

Name	Request

Results

_____

_____

_____

_____

_____

_____

better together in compassion

SCRIPTURE MEMORY VERSE
*This is what the LORD Almighty says: "Administer true justice;
show mercy and compassion to one another."*
ZECHARIAH 7:9

What does it mean to show true mercy and compassion to one another?
J. P. Kent, who is serving a life sentence without the possibility of parole,
became the grateful recipient of such when he was badly beaten by a
group of fellow inmates his first night in county jail. As he wrote in a
letter to his mother:

> Still wearing my bloody, dirty clothes, I looked for an open bunk.
> I finally found one and struggled to climb up onto it. . . One by
> one, at least ten different guys, all ages and races . . . began to
> place items on it. I tried to protest, but I could hardly move due
> to the pain. I watched canteen items they'd purchased individu-
> ally pile up on my bunk: a toothbrush, toothpaste, soap, de-
> odorant, a washcloth, gym shorts, a T-shirt, candy bars, paper, a
> pen. . . . I knew it was a real sacrifice for the men to give to me out
> of what little they had. I was shocked by their compassionate
> concern, and even more surprised by their generosity. They
> didn't know me and owed me nothing, yet they poured agape
> love all over me. I began to tear up from all the emotions within
> me. God used these maximum security prisoners to show me

what his grace and favor looked like. I definitely didn't earn or deserve it. . . . I was more vulnerable and needy than I'd ever been in my life, and these men took care of me that night. I felt like Jesus himself was ministering to me.[1]

This incident had a tremendous impact on J. P., who has now spent many years reaching out to other inmates with the same compassion, mercy and grace he received that first night.

Day 1

MERCY

Merciful God, every single day I live only under the gift of Your mercy. Thank you for not giving me what I deserve but offering me the compassion I don't deserve. Amen.

According to Zechariah 7:9, this week's memory verse, the Lord Almighty commands us to do what three things?

1. _____
2. _____
3. _____

What is the dictionary definition of "mercy"?

_____
_____
_____
_____

One way to understand mercy is to regard it as the act of God not giving us what we deserve. How does King David express this in Psalm 25:6-7?

_____
_____
_____
_____

When God hears our cries for mercy, how should we respond to Him (see Psalm 28:6-7)?

_____

_____

_____

According to Psalm 79:8, when do most people usually cry out to God for mercy?

_____

_____

_____

Do you know people who are in "desperate need" today? What would showing them mercy look like?

_____

_____

_____

_____

Whenever you show kindness to someone who is needy, what else are you doing (see Proverbs 14:31)?

_____

_____

_____

Read Luke 6:36. Why should we show mercy?

_____

_____

_____

_____

Lord, I need to be kind to everyone, even if I don't think they deserve it. Help me reach out with a gift of mercy to everyone I meet so You get the credit. Amen.

Day 2 COMFORT

*Father, I need You today because I feel a bit in need of compassion myself.
Thank You for promising to wrap me in Your arms of refuge. Amen.*

One way we reach out with compassion is to offer comfort. In the New
Testament, the Greek term most often used to convey this is *paraklesis*—
which has a double meaning of both encouragement and consolation. In
Handel's oratorio *Messiah,* perhaps one of the most beautiful refrains
contains the words of Isaiah 40:1. According to this verse, what does God
tell Isaiah to do?

_____

_____

_____

_____

Read Isaiah 40:2. What are some of the ways the people are comforted?

_____

_____

_____

_____

Read Psalm 22:24. What are the three things God did to comfort the
psalmist?

1. _____

2. _____

3. _____

Think of a time when someone comforted you. What did that look and
feel like?

_____

_____

_____

_____

Have you ever experienced comfort from God? Read Nahum 1:7. Why can you count on God as a source of comfort?

_____

_____

_____

_____

Comforting one another is an important aspect of being better together. Read 2 Corinthians 1:3-6. In verse 1, Paul mentions "the Father of compassion and the God of all comfort." According to verse 4, what does He do and why?

_____

_____

_____

_____

According to verse 5, where do we get what we need to comfort others?

_____

_____

_____

_____

Aside from being able to comfort someone in a similar situation, suffering through some trial also allows you to find some joy and sense in the suffering. Pastor Gene Getz experienced this in his own life:

> One time when I was disillusioned and in emotional turmoil, I studied the lives of Christians that God has used in special ways. As I read, I noticed a pattern. I saw that God often used suffering to eventually enable them to help others who were going through the same deep waters. That sudden insight changed my psychological disposition. It enabled me to experience joy in the midst of turmoil and to make sense out of what seemed chaotic.[2]

Have you ever suffered through something and later met someone undergoing a similar trial? How did your interaction with that person reflect Paul's words in verse 6?

_____
_____
_____
_____

God, when I needed Your comfort, You were there for me through the presence of others. From now on, when others need my comfort, help me to be Your comfort and compassion for them. Amen.

Day 3

JUSTICE

Awesome God, I want to do right and act justly, just as You require. But I need wisdom to know how to live that out in my world today. Thank You for hearing and providing as I know You will. Amen.

Read Micah 6:8. What does "act justly" mean?

_____
_____
_____
_____

In Psalm 106:3, we are called blessed if we act justly by doing what?

_____
_____
_____
_____

Isaiah 1:17 tells us to "learn to do right" by doing four things. Tell what each action is, and write down a practical way this could be put into practice. Put an asterisk by it if you have actually taken such an action.

Way to do right	Way to put into practice
1.	
2.	
3.	
4.	

New York City pastor Tim Keller notes the following on why justice should be important to every Christian:

> God's grace makes you just. The gospel is such that even though you're not saved by good works, you are saved by grace and faith—and it will change your life and lead to good works. . . . My definition of justice is giving humans their due as people in the image of God. We all agree that everyone deserves not to be enslaved, beaten, raped, or killed. We are not just talking about helping the poor, but helping people whose rights are being violated. . . . I want people to remember that the impetus for helping people comes from the experience of grace.[3]

Read Isaiah 30:18. How does justice go hand in hand with compassion?

_____

_____

_____

_____

Gracious God, You have continued to show me compassion,
even when I don't deserve your mercy. Please help me to act justly
toward others and reflect Your unfailing love toward me. Amen.

BURDENS

Dear Jesus, You know my burdens are getting heavy now, and I so long to lay them down. Help me to do so, knowing You will carry them for me. Amen.

Pilgrim's Progress, the classic Christian allegory written by John Bunyan in 1678, tells the story of an everyman named Christian who journeys through life, carrying a huge burden of sin on his back. As he travels from his hometown (the City of Destruction) to his final home (the Celestial City), he is constantly weighed down by this burden of sin. He has many adventures, but at the end of his journey, he comes upon a cross and begins to run toward it, still encumbered by his heavy weight:

> So I saw in my dream, that just as Christian came up to the cross, his burden loosed from off his shoulders, and fell from off his back, and began to tumble, and so continued to do till it came to the mouth of the sepulcher, where it fell in, and I saw it no more.[4]

Just as Christian was weighed down by his many sins and then released from them at the cross, so can we be free to live an unencumbered life. We can appropriate all Christ has done for us on the cross, where He took the punishment for our sins—all that burdens us. Do you have a lot of "burdens" that you carry around every day? What weighs you down heavily and perhaps keeps you from pursuing a fuller and freer life? (Think and pray about this before you write down your answer.)

What does Psalm 55:22 tell us to do with everything that concerns us and all of the burdens in our lives?

What will God do for us in return for our laying it all down at His feet?

_____

_____

_____

Peter also had some advice for those who are weighed down by worldly cares or a lifetime of regret. Read 1 Peter 5:6-7. What two things does he suggest we do?

1. _____

2. _____

What is God's part in all of this?

_____

_____

_____

As we allow God to lift our burdens, we must naturally move toward responding in kind to our fellow human beings. This is an important "one another" in the area of compassion. It's hard enough to try and carry our own burdens, but what radical command did Paul give in Galatians 6:2?

_____

_____

_____

What are some ways you can help carry someone else's burdens?

_____

_____

_____

_____

Father, it can be exhausting to help someone else in need by carrying his or her burdens. Yet I know this is the way to true compassion, so please give me open hands, strong shoulders and a willing heart. Amen.

Day 5 PEACE

Prince of Peace, bring peace to my heart, so I can calmly and deliberately move out in my community and beyond. I cannot do this alone, but You can help me. Amen.

Those who have compassion for other people usually rate peace as a high priority in their lives. In fact, we are called to be peacemakers. Read Colossians 3:15. From whom do we obtain an attitude of peace?

_____
_____
_____
_____

Why is an attitude of peace important for fellowship?

_____
_____
_____
_____

What is another quality of peace-loving people (see Colossians 3:15)?

_____
_____
_____
_____

Most of us have myriad relationships with all sorts of different people, and having an attitude of peace with all of them does not come naturally and is not easy. According to Titus 3:3, what are some of the behaviors that do seem to come naturally for us?

_____
_____
_____

According to Titus 3:4-5, what happened to change all these bad behaviors in our lives?

_____

_____

_____

_____

How has Jesus' saving grace changed you—what about your behavior has changed?

_____

_____

_____

_____

Read Titus 3:1-2. What seven good behaviors should those who are saved exhibit?

1. _____
2. _____
3. _____
4. _____
5. _____
6. _____
7. _____

According to Isaiah 32:17, those who seek to live a righteous life will exhibit what fruit?

_____

_____

_____

_____

_____

Read John 14:27. What does the peace that comes from Christ look like in a person's life?

_____

_____

_____

_____

Lord, the world does not know the kind of peace You offer, but I know that it would be a welcome commodity for those in turmoil. Help me to share Your peace with others. Amen.

Day
6

REFLECTION AND APPLICATION

God, You are my safe place and my strong tower. You alone know how many times I have run to You and been held and comforted. I will always need You and I depend on Your promise never to forsake me. Amen.

When you were a child, where (or to whom) did you go for comfort and compassion?

_____

_____

_____

_____

Today, where do you go for comfort and compassion?

_____

_____

_____

_____

_____

If your answer to the second question did not include God—your heavenly Father—close your eyes and picture yourself crawling up into His lap and allowing Him to hold you in His arms of love and care. What would you say to Him?

In *Flourish: Discover the Daily Joy of Abundant, Vibrant Living*, Catherine Hart Weber writes the following:

> God longs to be our ultimate safe haven; our source of comfort; a harbor to which we can turn when life's seas get rough; and a place where we can be loved, cared for, and protected. . . . He knows that His comfort is more fulfilling than any other's. . . . God is not only our safe haven, He is also our secure base. He provides a source of courage and confidence from which we can venture out into our daily living. Life is very complex. There are so many decisions to make, and we encounter major challenges almost daily. So we need both safety and security. We need to know that God is going before us, making a way and guiding us, and that He'll be there for us, available and supportive.[5]

When you daily meet with God for your quiet time together, aside from praising God and thanking Him and making requests of Him, do you also sit quietly and listen to Him? Do you listen for His direction? His guidance? What new thing could you do or what new place could you go to today if you truly felt that God was not only your compassionate refuge but also your guiding influence?

Savior, out of Your arms and into a needy world I go. Give me courage, strength, faith and power to accompany You in kingdom work. Amen.

REFLECTION AND APPLICATION

*Heavenly Father, You send angels to us all the time in the guise
of ordinary people. May we recognize that their compassion and
service come from You and for You. Amen.*

Remember J. P. Kent, the young inmate from earlier this week? Several
years into his life sentence, he wrote to his mother about yet another experience of mercy, this time when he was rushed to a hospital with a rup-
tured appendix. Because the authorities wouldn't tell his parents his
location, his mother couldn't be there to comfort her son's pain. But
God sent Nurse Betty:

> Nurse Betty not only did an excellent job of caring for me, but
> she acted as if I was her own son. She didn't hesitate to help me
> in ways that no other hospital staff member ever considered. She
> saw my needs, respected me as a human being who was suffer-
> ing, and provided tangible aid. . . . Experiencing those qualities
> in such an up-close-and-personal way was like having God as-
> sure me that I wasn't forgotten by Him—that I would be taken
> care of even though I was separated forever from daily life with
> my loved ones. In fact, Nurse Betty's agape love and merciful ac-
> tions were unlike anything I had experienced outside my own
> family in a very long time. . . . She was like "Jesus with skin on"
> to me during those five days in the hospital.[6]

Briefly describe a time when you have been "Jesus with skin on" for
someone—one of your children, a church member, a good friend, a
stranger you saw in need.

_____

_____

_____

_____

_____

We can all be "Jesus with skin on" to someone, and what we do can be as simple as giving a hug, providing a shoulder, or opening a door for someone whose hands are full. Be on the lookout for ways to show compassion for other people, and remember that you walk in His power.

Lord, make me an instrument of your peace.
Where there is hatred, let me sow love;
where there is injury, pardon;
where there is doubt, faith;
where there is despair, hope;
where there is darkness, light;
and where there is sadness, joy.

O Divine Master, grant that I may not so much seek to be
  consoled as to console;
to be understood as to understand;
to be loved, as to love.
For it is in giving that we receive;
it is in pardoning that we are pardoned;
and it is in dying that we are born to eternal life. Amen.[7]

Notes
1. Carol Kent, *Between a Rock and a Grace Place: Divine Surprises in the Tight Spots of Life* (Grand Rapids, MI: Zondervan Publishers, 2010), pp. 118-119.
2. Gene Getz, *Encouraging One Another,* One Another Series (Colorado Springs, CO: Victor Books, 2002), p. 162.
3. Kristen Scharold, "What We Owe the Poor," *Christianity Today* (December 2010), p. 69.
4. John Bunyan, *Pilgrim's Progress,* Section 3, quoted at *Internet Sacred Text Archive,* http://www.sacred-texts.com/chr/bunyan/pp03.htm (accessed April 2, 2011).
5. Catherine Hart Weber, *Flourish: Discover the Daily Joy of Abundant, Vibrant Living* (Minneapolis, MN: Bethany House Publishers, 2010), pp. 85-86.
6. Kent, *Between a Rock and a Grace Place,* p. 50.
7. This prayer has been attributed to Francis of Assisi.

Group Prayer Requests

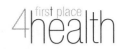

Today's Date: _____

Name	Request

Results

_____

_____

_____

_____

_____

_____

better together in encouragement

SCRIPTURE MEMORY VERSE

Encourage one another and build each other up, just as in fact you are doing.

I THESSALONIANS 5:11

If you've ever felt up against a brick wall, you will identify with Paul's challenges as he sought to follow God and lead the Early Church—he with the infamous reputation as a persecutor of Christians! It took an encouraging friend to pave the way for him to interact with the other believers. Barnabas, "Son of Encouragement," had a profound effect on bringing together community—as a bridge between the men who were called to be apostles while Christ was on earth and the man who was called to be an apostle after Christ had returned to heaven (see Acts 4:36).

Read Acts 9:26-27. How did Barnabas encourage others to accept Paul?

_____

_____

_____

Now read Acts 11:22-23. How did Barnabas continue to encourage the Early Church far and wide?

_____

_____

_____

_____

Day
1

BUILD

Dear Lord, thank You for building me up through Your love. May I, in turn, seek to build up others through my encouragement. Amen.

In this week's memory verse, 1 Thessalonians 5:11, encouraging one another is described as building each other up. What does it mean to "build up?"

_____

_____

_____

_____

What does it mean to "tear down" another person?

_____

_____

_____

_____

We are called to do just the opposite of tearing down! Yet if we are not consciously seeking to build up other people, then perhaps we are having an adverse effect on them. What is the warning given to us in Hebrews 3:13?

_____

_____

_____

_____

What is something you could do daily to encourage another person?

_____

_____

_____

_____

_____

In Romans 14:19, what two tangible results of our efforts to be encouraging are suggested by the apostle Paul?

1. _____

2. _____

"To spur on" is similar to "build up," and Hebrews 10:24 tells us two objectives to have as we encourage others. What are they?

1. _____

2. _____

Father of compassion, may I never use my words to tear someone down but always to spur them on toward You and Your way. Amen.

SPEAK Day 2

God, You are the Word and the giver of words. May I choose wisely what words come out of my mouth and are heard by others. Amen.

The word "encourage" means to inspire courage in someone who needs it. And who doesn't need it? The right word of affirmation spoken at the right time can offer another person the courage he or she needs to take important and meaningful steps in life. The timing of our words is important. What observation is made in Proverbs 25:11, and why is this true?

_____

_____

_____

Read Proverbs 12:25. What does a kind word do?

_____

_____

_____

According to Proverbs 16:24, what are some of the other benefits of pleasant words to another person?

_____

_____

_____

When has someone spoken a word of encouragement when you felt saddened by or worried about something?

_____

_____

_____

C. S. Lewis once said, "Friendship is born at that moment when one person says to another: 'What! You too! I thought I was the only one.'" Sharing words of encouragement shows others that they are not alone. Have you ever felt as if you were the only one who has experienced a particular problem? If so, how has your fellowship with other First Place 4 Health members or with people in your church helped you to see that you are not alone?

_____

_____

_____

_____

Thank You, God, for Your Word, which is a healing balm to my soul. Help me to know it and use it to encourage others toward healing and health. Amen.

Day 3 WATCH

Open my eyes, Lord, that I may see and understand what others are going through in order to seek out ways to help them, through Your power. Amen.

There is no way we can encourage someone else unless we are aware of their lives—their day-to-day activities, struggles, challenges and feelings.

We need to be involved and to listen actively and, yes, even to ask the hard questions sometimes. In general, encouraging words communicate the thought, *I know who you are; I care about you,* and *I'm here to help you.* According to Acts 13:15, what were Paul and his companions told to do to help the people?

_____

_____

_____

_____

When we are aware of others' needs, we are acting in what way, according to 1 Thessalonians 2:11?

_____

_____

_____

_____

According to 1 Thessalonians 2:12, in what three tangible ways are we to show our care and concern?

1. _____

2. _____

3. _____

It's hard to keep being an encourager sometimes, isn't it? Often there is no response from the other person, or we don't see the change we had hoped for. According to Psalm 10:17, what does the Lord do for everyone, including those of us who are reaching out?

_____

_____

_____

_____

Sometimes the best way to encourage one another is to listen, not talk. Like God, we become aware of those around us when we actively "listen to their cry" and truly hear what they are saying (also perhaps reading between the lines to surmise what they are not saying). Watching a person's reaction to our words might help us realize when we need to be quiet. Radio personality and First Place 4 Health author Christin Ditchfield talks about cultivating this trait:

> Sometimes we're in too much of a hurry to "fix" things and make them better. It's a trap I've fallen into. Many times I've caught myself trying to solve friends' problems by offering what I intend to be helpful suggestions. "Have you thought of this? Have you tried that? Maybe if you just. . . . " Often they will shoot down one idea after another: They have a million reasons why nothing I tell them will work. And still I keep trying, instead of getting the message: "I need your sympathy, not your solutions. A listening ear; not a list of things to do." I don't know why I'm so slow to pick up on this—especially considering how frustrating I find it when other people do it to me. I guess I really do just want to help, the same way others want to help me. But years ago, I learned to tell my friends and family up front "I may ask you for advice about this later; right now I just need you to listen."[1]

Have you ever offered what you thought were practical ways to solve a problem, only to have your ideas brushed aside and a different solution used? How did you react? What would you do differently next time?

_____

_____

_____

_____

Have you ever been offered solutions to a problem when what you really needed was a good listener? How did you handle the situation? How would you do things differently if it happens again, or would you do the same thing?

_____

_____

_____

_____

_____

> *Oh Father, I need to be more alert to what's going on in the lives of the people around me. Help me to be more watchful and aware. Help me to discern when others need my words or my ear. Amen.*

ADMONISH   Day 4

> *Almighty God, please guide me to reach out in encouragement and love when I have to say hard things. Amen.*

While encouragement is a positive action, there are aspects of it that can often be challenging—especially those times when we must care enough to say hard things to another person. The word "admonish" can mean both to rebuke somebody mildly but earnestly and to advise somebody not to do something. According to 2 Timothy 4:2, what are believers reminded to always be prepared to do?

_____

_____

_____

_____

What two important qualities must we display when we admonish, or rebuke, someone?

1. _____

2. _____

Why do you think there is so much emphasis on our own manner when we admonish someone?

_____

_____

_____

_____

According to 1 Thessalonians 5:14, what kind of admonition is necessary for each of the four groups of people?

1. _____

2. _____

3. _____

4. _____

What would happen if we tried to admonish someone, but we didn't first pray and carefully prepare what to say?

_____

_____

_____

Read Acts 20:31. How do you know that Paul felt intensely about warning the new church not to be led astray?

_____

_____

_____

_____

Sometimes our admonishment can be misinterpreted. According to 1 Corinthians 4:14, what was Paul *not* doing when he admonished?

_____

_____

_____

Have you ever had to admonish someone? Did you pray and prepare ahead of time? How did the person react to what you had to say?

_____

_____

_____

Lord, please give me wisdom to know when admonishment is necessary and gentleness in my words when I rebuke or advise someone. Amen.

PERSEVERE Day 5

God, my strength and shield, truly You are the One who keeps me going when I feel like giving up. Help me to persevere to the end and glorify You in the process. Amen.

It's not always easy to encourage others and speak the truth. Acts 14 records how Paul was stoned for doing that, but when he recovered, he and Barnabas continued on their missionary journey of encouragement. According to Acts 14:22, what were their two guiding passions?

1. _____

2. _____

Perseverance is needed in order to remain true to the faith. In fact, in verse 22, what did Paul and Barnabas say about this?

_____

_____

_____

What is the reason for perseverance stated in Hebrews 10:36?

_____

_____

_____

What has God promised to those who persevere in doing His will?

_____

_____

_____

Followers of Christ will face challenging times and be tempted to give up. What might make someone feel like giving up on the journey toward more balanced health?

_____

_____

_____

What would encourage a person not to give up the journey?

_____

_____

_____

_____

Read James 1:2-4. What do verses 2-3 say we should do when we experience trials?

_____

_____

_____

What is the result of perseverance mentioned in verse 4?

_____

_____

_____

_____

Lord, no one enjoys being tested by trials, but if that is the path to being a person who sticks it out over the long haul, then I'm ready. It is You who give me strength, and with You by my side, I can do anything. Amen.

REFLECTION AND APPLICATION

Lord, truly Your love is the greatest gift I have ever received, and I know that I don't deserve it. Help me show others that they too are loved by You. Amen.

Perhaps the best words of encouragement any of us will ever hear are "God loves you." Henri Nouwen once said, "The best gift my friendship can give to you is the gift of your Belovedness."[2] Each of us is the beloved of God, but often our encouragement is needed to help others claim and realize their own belovedness. Then each of us can learn to recognize the voice of love that speaks into our hearts and to tune out all other voices who try to define us by their approval or disapproval. As Stephen Smith writes:

> When we speak to each other, reminding one another of our uniqueness and our belovedness, we come to realize that we do offer something no one else offers. This is why reminding and affirming one another of being the beloved is so vitally important.
>
> Community is the place where this should happen. In our competitive workplaces, schools, and world, we won't hear much talk about love. These are the places where the language of being the beloved competes with the language of earned acceptance. Our various communities—healthy families; safe friendships; churches—are where we look forward to being accepted, embraced, touched, and recognized for who we are.[3]

Why is the world's approval or disapproval not as important as God's?

Why are you beloved by God?

How does the First Place 4 health program encourage your uniqueness and belovedness?

_____

_____

_____

Thank You, Father, for unconditional love and acceptance that defines me. I no longer choose to be defined by the world's approval, only as Your beloved.

Day 7 REFLECTION AND APPLICATION

Father, how thankful I am to You for those times when You use even me to speak a living word into someone's life. Amen.

What can we do when we don't know what to say and words of encouragement don't come easily? What are some resources that have helped you to know how and what to speak as encouragement to someone?

_____

_____

_____

_____

Our most important source should, of course, be the Bible. As Christin Ditchfield states:

> As we continue to seek God's guidance on how to encourage others, we must always remember to base our words on the Word of God. In a time of crisis, in a moment of need, when someone comes to us with a problem, when we can see that someone is headed for danger or disaster, it's often our opportunity and our privilege to speak into their lives, to pierce through the darkness and confusion, and to point them to the Light. Sometimes it's a

special, one-time occurrence—a "divine appointment" of sorts; with others, we'll have the opportunity over and over again. . . . Often we can draw on our own experiences—our failures as well as our successes. . . . But most important are the things God has taught us in the pages of his Word, the biblical principles that are the foundation of our life and faith. . . . We can be prepared by making sure we spend time daily in God's presence, studying his Word, seeking his face, asking him to give us His wisdom—to fill us with it—so that whenever we need it, it's there.[4]

Reading the Bible and studying Scripture will prepare you for so many things in life and provide you with many stories and truths that you can use to encourage others (and yourself of course!). You should have memorized by now six verses of Scripture. Of those six, which has been of particular help and encouragement for you? Why?

_____

_____

_____

_____

Dear God, You know my heart and You know what my days are like.
Sometimes I really need to hear encouragement, especially when I feel as if
I'm lagging behind in some way. Help me overflow with Your love so that
I can encourage other people, because I know that when I encourage others,
I also encourage myself—especially when I use Your Word. You are so great,
and I am so thankful that You think of me as Your beloved. Amen.

Notes

1. Christin Ditchfield, *A Way with Words: What Women Should Know About the Power They Possess* (Wheaton, IL: Crossway Books, 2010), pp. 49-50.
2. Stephen W. Smith, *Embracing Soul Care: Making Space for What Matters Most* (Grand Rapids, MI: Kregel Publishers, 2006), p. 59.
3. Ibid., p. 60.
4. Ditchfield, *A Way with Words,* pp. 44-45.

Group Prayer Requests

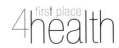

Today's Date: _____

Name	Request

Results

_____

_____

_____

_____

_____

_____

better together in
harmony

SCRIPTURE MEMORY VERSE
*Finally, all of you, live in harmony with one another; be sympathetic,
love as brothers, be compassionate and humble.*
1 PETER 3:8

What does it mean to live in harmony with one another? The term "harmony" is derived from the Greek word *harmonia,* which means concord, joint or agreement. It is also related to the Greek verb *harmozo,* which means to join or fit together. Although these terms are most often used in connection with music and the arts, they certainly form a good description of what the Body of Christ should be. In ancient Greece, *harmonia* was used to describe a combination of contrasting elements—the employment at the same time of both higher and lower notes. Putting together these different elements made something harmonious—a sound that pleases.

LIKE-MINDEDNESS

Day 1

Heavenly Father, thank You for creating us to be different and yet able to work together in harmony, like-minded in our love for You and each other, to produce a living music that will touch the world. Amen.

When we seek harmony with others—even others quite different from ourselves—we become a pleasing and harmonious group. The challenge is, of course, how can we do that?

According to this week's memory verse, 1 Peter 3:8, what are four ways we can begin to live in harmony with one another?

1. _____
2. _____
3. _____
4. _____

Which of these is the hardest for you to do when in a large group? Why?

_____
_____
_____
_____

Sometimes it is hard to make a "pleasing sound" when we are with those who have different backgrounds, worldviews, values and socioeconomic levels. Because we have many differences, we have a tendency to gravitate toward those who (at least for the most important life issues or concerns) think the same as we do. In your First Place 4 Health group, what two interests do all of the members have in common—in what ways are you like-minded?

1. _____
2. _____

God created us to be unique, and He gives us different gifts to offer to the Body. However, on some non-negotiables, we are encouraged to be like-minded. According to Philippians 2:2, what does Paul say these areas are?

_____
_____
_____
_____

Yet if we all only sang the same note in the same way all of the time, there would be no musical harmony. So what should we do in regard to people who are different from us (see Romans 12:16)?

_____

_____

_____

What does Paul say we should not do in regard to ourselves?

_____

_____

_____

Dear God, please help me reinforce those areas I have in common with others and focus on the positive in my relationships. Amen.

BELONGING — Day 2

Lord, please help me to know that I do belong somewhere and have a distinct role to play in an important story that You are crafting. Amen.

"I wouldn't want to belong to any club that would have me as a member." So said Groucho Marx in an attempt to be funny—or at least to ward off exclusivity in advance. The truth is, we all want to belong somewhere—to be accepted and received. In fact, it is when we belong that we are the happiest:

> New scientific research has borne out the fact that when comparing extremely happy people with average happy people, the one characteristic that made the difference is meaningful, lasting, relationship attachments. Those who have a broad range of social connections, with generations of families living close together, have the highest happiness. The neurobiology of attachments explains that healthy relationship connections stimulate

the brain activity that helps to create systems that lead to our developing empathy and enjoyment of positive interactions, and managing stress that goes with negative interactions.[1]

Do you have a lot of different friends and relatives with whom you are in close contact? If so, how do these relationships add to your sense of belonging?

_____

_____

_____

In Paul's wonderful chapter of Romans 12, he teaches that "in Christ we who are many form one body, and each member belongs to all the others" (verse 5). We are family! So if you think that you don't have a lot of friends and relatives you're close to, you *do* have family nearby! Read Romans 12:3-21. How does Paul compare the Body of Christ with the human body (see verses 4-5)?

_____

_____

_____

Paul lists many rules for living in harmony with others—how to be better together (see verses 9-21). Which of these rules is the hardest one for you to follow? Why?

_____

_____

_____

Why is it important that we who belong to the Body of Christ follow all of these rules?

_____

_____

_____

Read Romans 14:8 and John 15:19. If you ever felt as if you don't feel you belong somewhere, how can these passages reassure you?

_____

_____

_____

Dear God, sometimes I feel as if I don't fit in, as if I don't belong anywhere or with anyone. I know, though, that I belong to You and that I have a First Place family. Thank You for choosing me. Amen.

BODY

Day 3

Lord, I realize that You need all the parts of the Body of Christ to work together. Help me to know that my unique contribution is important. Amen.

Read 1 Corinthians 12:12-26. In this selection, Paul reminds us that "there should be no division in the body" (verse 25). What should each part do (see verses 25-26)?

_____

_____

_____

Why are God's people called a body, and why did He create us to be different (see verses 14-20)?

_____

_____

_____

Do you ever feel as if you are an unnecessary part of the Body of Christ? How does God encourage the unique importance of every one of His creations (see verses 21-24)?

_____

_____

_____

Our bodies and souls are so intertwined that what we feel in one area of our lives affects every other area of our lives. Because we are part of a larger Body, what we feel can then affect *that* Body. Read Proverbs 15:30 and 16:24. What can heal us?

_____

_____

_____

_____

Both our physical bodies and the fellowship of the Body of Christ need godly encouragement and support. In what way is one area of your life affecting the other areas today (for good or for ill)?

_____

_____

_____

_____

God who heals, please touch my human body with Your power so that I may use it to glorify You and bring about reconciliation and restoration to others. I want my body to be a healthy and active part of Your Body. Amen.

Day 4

UNITY

Dear Jesus, I want to work with other members of Your Body so that we act as one body with the sole purpose of furthering Your kingdom here on earth as it is in heaven. Amen.

We cannot *make* unity happen in a group of people, but each of us is responsible for doing our own part to help that unity happen. Read Ephesians 4:3-6. What unites all Christians?

_____

_____

_____

Why is it important that this unity not be disturbed?

_____

_____

_____

_____

Read Psalm 133. To what does the psalmist compare unity?

_____

_____

_____

_____

What does God do when the Body lives in unity (see verse 3)?

_____

_____

_____

_____

According to Romans 15:5-7, why are we called to unity?

_____

_____

_____

_____

Read John 17:23. In addition to glorifying God and bringing Him praise, what is another result of our unity in the eyes of a watching world?

_____

_____

_____

_____

Father, I know the world is watching me and other believers and I pray that what they see is a devoted Christ-follower who loves and serves. Amen.

ACCORD

*Father, rather than being a peacekeeper, may I become a peacemaker and
rely on You for power to leave a peaceful presence in my wake. Amen.*

Previously, we discussed how peace is the natural outcome of a life lived
in harmony with other people and how God calls us to be people of
peace. Strife and division was an issue in many of the early churches.
Look up 1 Corinthians 3:1-4. What does Paul mean when he says that
the believers are still not ready for "solid food"?

_____

_____

_____

_____

What is causing their setbacks (see verses 3-4)?

_____

_____

_____

_____

Earlier, in 1 Corinthians 1:10-15, Paul shed some light as to the source
of the division in the church. What was causing discord in this congregation? Does this type of issue still cause discord in the Church today?
In what ways?

_____

_____

_____

_____

What appeal did Paul make to the believers in verse 10?

_____

_____

_____

What does Paul mean when he asks, "Is Christ divided" (verse 13)?

_____

_____

_____

_____

What does James 4:1-2 state is often the source of fights and quarrels? What are we focusing on instead of God?

_____

_____

_____

_____

According to 2 Timothy 2:23-24, how are we to avoid divisions among us? Why is this often difficult to do?

_____

_____

_____

_____

Lord, help me to always focus on You and seek to bring peace to every situation. Help me to live in accord with those around me. Amen.

REFLECTION AND APPLICATION

Day 6

Jesus, You spent time with a variety of people. Help me to reach out to others in that way, even when it pushes me out of my comfort zone. Amen.

Do you see much unity and harmony in the Church today? Too often denominations divide over dogma, congregations draw lines based on social demographics, and individual Christians ignore the longing for unity that flows from the inner life of God. Dr. Timothy Jones, author and seminary professor, addressed how to regain true unity:

In order to recapture the truth that we need each other and we need the full variety of Christ's creation, one pastor remarked, "I've no desire to join a church filled with people 'just like me.' If everyone's educational level, economic status, and racial profile were similar to mine, why would we need each other? When I worship and pray with my Christian family, I long to be surrounded by a congregation that's as multicultural as an Eskimo drinking kosher vodka from a Mason jar. I want to sing the "Gloria Patri" back-to-back with "We Shall Overcome," "I'll Fly Away," and a string of rollicking praise choruses. I want to shake brown hands and white hands, smooth hands and calloused hands, wrinkled hands and tiny, trembling, newborn hands. Why? Because church is not about my personal tastes or desires. In fact, church is not about me at all. It is about a mismatched community of recovering sinners, bound by a Spirit that no one has ever seen."[2]

What can you do to promote harmony and unity in each of the following places?

Your *Better Together* study group

_____

_____

_____

_____

_____

Your family

_____

_____

_____

_____

_____

Your workplace

_____

_____

_____

_____

_____

Your neighborhood

_____

_____

_____

_____

Your community

_____

_____

_____

_____

Dear God, thank You for creating all of us in Your image. May I never forget that about everyone I meet, and may I treat those individuals with honor and respect that reflects Your glory. Help me to reach out to and accept people who are different from me so that our unity of belief and our harmony will draw others toward You. Amen.

REFLECTION AND APPLICATION

Day 7

Jesus, I could live a peaceful life if it weren't for all those other people out there! Seriously, I ask that You would help me to be peaceful inside and let that peace spill over to others. Amen.

As representatives of the Prince of Peace, we are told, "If it is possible, as far as it depends on you, live at peace with everyone " (Romans 12:18). In his book *Restoring Broken Things,* singer and author Steven Curtis Chapman points out the following:

> To live peaceably means that we seek to bring the shalom, or the peace of God, into relationships. A shalom-ed relationship is one in which there is order—that is, alignment, health, integration, celebration—just the way God designed relationships to be. Notice the two important qualifications Paul makes. First, he says to live peaceably with all, so far as it depends on you. Each of us must make the initiative in peacemaking and take responsibility for ourselves in all of our relationships. We are to be peacemakers "as unto the Lord," not making our obedience contingent on anyone's response. But Paul also instructs us to live peaceably with all, if possible. There may be unwillingness from the other party(ies) to engage in restoration. In these situations, the peacemaker must settle for the "peace" that he has done everything within his power to work for reconciliation and restoration.[3]

In general, when harmony and peace in a relationship are disturbed, what are some steps you can take to restore the relationship?

_____

_____

_____

_____

Think and pray about a relationship in your life, one in dire need of harmony, peace and restoration. What have you done to seek peace in that relationship?

_____

_____

_____

_____

How and when will you know that it's time to leave the results in God's hands and move on?

_____

_____

_____

_____

_____

> *God, grant me the serenity to accept the things I cannot change;*
> *courage to change the things I can; and wisdom to know the difference.*
> *Living one day at a time; enjoying one moment at a time; accepting*
> *hardships as the pathway to peace; taking, as He did, this sinful world*
> *as it is, not as I would have it; trusting that He will make all things right if I*
> *surrender to His Will; that I may be reasonably happy in this life and*
> *supremely happy with Him forever in the next. Amen.*[4]

Notes

1. C. R. Snyder and Shane J. Lopez, *Positive Psychology: The Scientific and Practical Explorations of Human Strengths* (Thousand Oaks, CA: Sage Publications, 2007).
2. Timothy Paul Jones, "What Does Jesus Want?" *Discipleship Journal* (March/April 2007), p. 33.
3. Steven Curtis Chapman and Scotty Smith, *Restoring Broken Things: What Happens When We Catch a Vision of the New World Jesus Is Creating* (Nashville, TN: Integrity Publishers, 2005), p. 133.
4. This prayer is at least partially attributed to Reinhold Niebuhr.

Group Prayer Requests

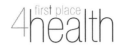

Today's Date: _____

Name	Request

Results

_____

_____

_____

_____

_____

better together in forgiveness

SCRIPTURE MEMORY VERSE

Bear with each other and forgive whatever grievances you may have against one another. Forgive as the Lord forgave you.

COLOSSIANS 3:13

Someone once said that "forgiveness is giving up your right to hurt someone back." Are you willing to give up that right? God's Word (and our week's memory verse) clearly states that we are to forgive one another, and the reason is that God has so graciously forgiven us.

Based on research on forgiveness, Dr. Everett Worthington Jr. explains the complexity of two different kinds of forgiveness: Decisional forgiveness is when we decide to forgive. Emotional forgiveness is when we are able to experience positive emotions in place of negative unforgiving emotions. We don't always experience both kinds of forgiveness. For instance, we may decide to forgive a drunk driver who caused a death but still not feel warmly toward that person.[1] It is within our power to choose to forgive, and the results are always for our benefit.

GRIEVANCES

Day 1

Heavenly Father, I've been carrying too much stuff—too many complaints—around, and I so want to let go of it all in order to move forward with You in freedom. Please help me. Amen.

Have you ever kept a list of grudges against someone else? Perhaps you haven't actually written them down, but in your mind, the list grows every time another incident occurs. The Bible calls these "grievances" and specifically says that we are to forgive them. Read Luke 7:44-50, a story about a sinful woman who came to Jesus. What did the woman do to indicate that she wanted to be forgiven?

_____

_____

_____

What did Jesus say to her? What saved her?

_____

_____

_____

If we truly understand that it was our sins that Jesus took to the cross, then how can we refuse to let go of our tightly held grudges? Read Job 31:13-15. Why did Job forgive others' grievances?

_____

_____

_____

_____

If a person carries grievances deep inside, how do those grievances affect the relationship with the person or those people who caused the pain?

_____

_____

_____

_____

How might the relationship influence how a person relates to other people in general?

_____

_____

_____

In *Essentials for Life*, Marcia Ford states that "Studies have shown that forgiving people enjoy good health and well-being, have lower blood pressure and stronger immune systems, and experience fewer stress-related disorders and less cardiovascular disease. The benefits have been proven to be so dramatic that it is in your own best interest to develop a forgiving nature."[2] How has your health or the health of someone you know been affected by holding on to a grievance?

_____

_____

_____

_____

Today you might want to spend some time in prayer before the Lord with open hands, letting go of any and all grudges.

> *Here I am, Father, with open hands and open heart, laying at Your feet all my grudges and grievances so that You can handle them in Your way and Your time. Help me to live a healthy life balanced in all ways. Thank You. Amen.*

REPENTANCE   Day 2

> *Forgive me, Lord, for too often choosing to go my way and not Yours, for doing my will and not Yours. Thank You for offering me a fresh start and a direction for my life every day. Amen.*

Repentance means to make a 180-degree turn and begin to go in the opposite direction. For a sinner, this is how the forgiveness process starts. We must first recognize that we have chosen to go our way and not God's way, and then we confess that sin to our Savior and ask for His forgiveness. According to 1 John 1:9, what two things will happen when we confess our sins?

1. _____

2. _____

Why does God do those things?

_____

_____

_____

Repentance leads not only to blessing but also to power. What did Peter ask the crowds to do on the Day of Pentecost, and what was the result (see Acts 2:38-41)?

_____

_____

_____

_____

Read Mark 1:15. What does "the kingdom of God has come near" mean, and why should that encourage people to repent?

_____

_____

_____

According to Ezekiel 18:21, what must a person do in order to live and not die?

_____

_____

_____

What extra benefit will there be (see Ezekiel 18:22)?

_____

_____

_____

_____

Oh, God of mercy and grace, thank You for remembering my sins no more and allowing me to walk forward in forgiveness and new life. Amen.

REDEMPTION

Day
3

Lord, You have called me by name and redeemed me. That is an incredible thought, and I am filled with awesome wonder just to realize it. Amen.

What promise did the Lord give to His people (see Isaiah 43:1)?

_____

_____

_____

What is the dictionary definition of "redeemed"?

_____

_____

_____

In my dictionary, the first definition is "to make something acceptable or pleasant in spite of its negative qualities and aspects," and the third definition is "to pay for the sins of humanity with Jesus Christ's death on the cross." How do these two definitions relate to each other and to us?

_____

_____

_____

What aspect of God's character offers us this redemption (see Ephesians 1:7)?

_____

_____

_____

In 1 Peter 1:18-21, Peter wrote as a person who fully knew about the need to be redeemed. With what does the world redeem things?

_____

_____

_____

From what were we redeemed (see verse 18)?

_____

_____

_____

What is the result of our redemption (see verse 21)?

_____

_____

_____

> *Lord, that You can take someone such as me and fashion and make me fit for Your use in the Kingdom is true redemption. Thank You from the bottom of my heart for Your forgiveness. Amen.*

Day 4

PROCESS

Father, I want to be a person who willingly forgives others. Work in my heart and in my life so that I can extend grace and mercy to all around me. Amen.

Sometimes forgiveness is a process that takes time, with the process itself being as important as the forgiveness. No one said anything in life would be easy, but the process of forgiveness is essential for a life of health and a healthy faith. What is the greatest benefit of our forgiving others (see Matthew 6:14)?

_____

_____

_____

Saul was the number one persecutor of Christians, yet on the road to Damascus, God appeared to him and changed his life. Read Acts 26:12-18. What did the voice from heaven say to Saul?

_____

_____

_____

What was the process Paul went through to be forgiven?

_____

_____

_____

In the process of forgiving others, we must take the first step and leave the ultimate consequences of others' sins where (see Proverbs 20:22)?

_____

_____

_____

Even a person like Peter, who was forgiven much, wondered how long such a process could last. Read Matthew 18:21-22. What did Peter ask Jesus, and what was Jesus' response?

_____

_____

_____

If you are in the middle of the process of forgiving someone, ask God to help you stay the course for the end result of your own freedom.

O Lord, You have requested that I continue to forgive and forgive and forgive. How could I do any less, since You have forgiven me so much? Amen.

FREEDOM — Day 5

God, I want to let go and allow You to take over all the hurt and pain that I have been carrying around for so long. I know this is the only path to true freedom. Amen.

When we forgive, "we set a prisoner free and discover that the prisoner is us."[3] This statement by Dr. Lewis Smedes speaks eloquently of the simple truth that God wants to free us from the bonds of shame, resentment and bitterness. Do you want to live freely? Then follow the admonition given in this week's memory verse—forgive one another. How does the image in Luke 6:38 symbolize what our life can be like if we take that first gracious and giving step toward forgiveness?

_____

_____

_____

In Romans 6:6, Paul refers to us as "slaves to sin." What happened to free us from this slavery (see Romans 6:7)?

_____

_____

_____

Read Romans 6:14-18. Paul said that we change "masters." Who did we obey in the past, and what authority are we under now?

_____

_____

_____

When you take steps on the journey of forgiveness, remember that God is with you and He will both lead the process and usher you into new freedom and health on all levels.

> *Lord, on this journey toward balanced health, forgiveness is a major*
> *advance for me physically, spiritually, emotionally and mentally.*
> *Thank You for prodding me in this direction. Amen.*

Day 6 REFLECTION AND APPLICATION

> *Lord, Please cleanse me and spur me to have a positive and forgiving attitude*
> *toward others so that they may see Christ in me. Amen.*

Dr. Catherine Hart Weber warns about some of the ramifications of holding on to grievances:

When we hold on to anger and resentment, it leads to ruminating on our offenses. . . . Bitterness and resentment take root and create a grudge. . . . Holding a grudge poisons all your life systems, causes you to languish, and can even make you sick. That is because it increases the level of stress hormones, blood pressure, hostility, and the chance of depression along with the desire to numb and soothe your pain with shopping, food, and substances. Holding a grudge can cause you to redefine a part of your life by how you have been hurt. . . .

Letting go of grudges releases all your life systems from excessive stress hormones and frees you to greater spiritual and psychological well-being. Forgiveness is the only way to heal yourself and free and repair relationships. When you let go of grudges, you have more freedom, health, happiness, and well-being.[4]

Have you ever not forgiven someone and have that unforgiveness lead you to soothe your pain by doing something you later regretted doing? What did you do?

_____

_____

_____

_____

Did you actually feel better, or did the pain come back to haunt you?

_____

_____

_____

Is the situation still unresolved? Do you still need to forgive? What good can come by holding on to something that you know is bad for you?

_____

_____

_____

In the future, how do you plan to handle situations when someone hurts you?

_____

_____

_____

_____

Jesus, at the cross You let go of everything and submitted to Your Father's will. Today I do the same. Have Your own way with me. Amen.

Day 6

REFLECTION AND APPLICATION

O God, even as I take steps to forgive others, I realize my actions may or may not affect them at all. But help me to move forward in truth and trust, regardless of their response. Amen.

"Unforgiveness is the poison we drink while hoping others will die." Sounds crazy, doesn't it? Who in the world would ever intentionally do that? Well, all too often we are the ones drinking that poison. Whenever we hold tightly to an unforgiving spirit, we are slowly dying to truth and righteousness.

While we are commanded to forgive, we must understand what forgiving does and does not involve. Steven Curtis Chapman states some truths that may help us in this area:

- Forgiving is not forgetting or ignoring an offense.
- Forgiving is not excusing, justifying, or pardoning an offense.
- Forgiving is not smothering a conflict.
- Forgiving is not tolerating what should not be tolerated.
- Forgiving does not always result in reconciliation.
- Forgiving does not mean you stop hurting.
- Forgiving is refusing to punish.

- Forgiving is a commitment not to repeat or discuss the matter with others.
- Forgiving is a radical commitment to uproot any residual bitterness.
- Forgiving is a choice to be merciful as God your Father has been merciful with you.[5]

Are there still some people who you need to forgive? Picture yourself kneeling at the feet of Jesus and carefully laying each grievance at His feet. Pray a prayer for each person as you let go of each grievance, and leave the consequences in His capable hands. Then never pick up the grievances again.

Dear God, You offer me freedom and forgiveness and I gladly accept them. Help me to be as generous with other people as You are with me. I don't really want to wallow in self-pity, but sometimes I find myself holding on to a grievance as if it were a flag I can wave in someone's face. Help me to forgive; help me to let go and move on in good grace. Help me to show those around me just how great You are. Amen.

Notes

1. Everett L. Worthington Jr., *A Just Forgiveness: Responsible Healing Without Excusing Injustice* (Downers Grove, IL: InterVarsity Press, 2009), p. 74.
2. Marcia Ford, *Essentials for Life: Your Back-to-Basics Guide to What Matters Most* (Nashville, TN: Thomas Nelson Publishers, 2010), p. 112.
3. Lewis B. Smedes, *The Art of Forgiving: When You Need to Forgive and Don't Know How* (New York: Ballantine Books, 1997), p. 178.
4. Catherine Hart Weber, *Flourish: Discover the Daily Joy of Abundant, Vibrant Living* (Minneapolis, MN: Bethany House Publishers, 2010), p. 118.
5. Steven Curtis Chapman and Scotty Smith, *Restoring Broken Things: What Happens When We Catch a Vision of the New World Jesus Is Creating* (Nashville, TN: Integrity Publishers, 2005), p. 134.

Group Prayer Requests

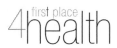

Today's Date: _____

Name	Request

Results

_____
_____
_____
_____
_____
_____

better together in honor

SCRIPTURE MEMORY VERSE

Be devoted to one another in brotherly love. Honor one another above yourselves.
ROMANS 12:10

What does the word "honor" mean to you? Perhaps the first thing that comes to mind is a school's honor code. A school's honor code outlines the standards of an educational community. If an individual doesn't live by the code, they are disciplined and sometimes even cast out from the community. This concept of honor was passed down through the ages. Medieval knights were obliged to give mercy if their opponent yielded in battle. And men were honor bound to confront one another when challenged in a duel. What are some modern examples of being honor bound?

_____

_____

_____

_____

REVERENCE

Day 1

Heavenly Father, I know that life is not all about me, but obviously I have a vested interest in what goes on around me. Help me look out for others first.

According to Romans 12:10, our memory verse for this week, we are to honor others above ourselves. This means that we are to treat others as more important than we are. This is increasingly difficult to do in our "me first" culture. However, as Pastor Rick Warren began his bestselling book *The Purpose Driven Life*, "It's not about you." This clear statement set the whole tone for a practical book that elevates living to glorify God as the ultimate purpose of life. Read Proverbs 14:31, 20:3 and Ephesians 5:21. How do we show honor to God?

_____
_____
_____
_____
_____

According to Titus 2:3, how should men and women live?

_____
_____
_____
_____
_____

Sometimes we see people prospering who don't honor or show respect to anyone. According to Ecclesiastes 8:12, who will ultimately be better off?

_____
_____
_____
_____

What is one way you can show reverence to another person today?

_____
_____
_____
_____

What is one way you can show reverence to God today?

_____

_____

_____

_____

May I, Lord, be a person of honor. May I honor and glorify You first, and then may I honor those around me, in an effort to be a witness to Your name.

FAMILY

Day 2

Father above, please help me to honor those in my earthly family, regardless of how they treat me. Amen.

Honoring one another includes honoring members of our own families. This is not just a suggestion; it is a biblical command. Unfortunately, this is sometimes the hardest of all commands to follow. Each family has issues and brings together myriad personalities—people who might never choose to cross paths but, because they're related by blood, they sometimes must. Read Exodus 20:12 and Deuteronomy 5:16. What are we commanded to do?

_____

_____

_____

_____

What benefit do we receive when we follow this command?

_____

_____

_____

_____

According to Matthew 15:4, what should happen to anyone who curses their parents?

_____

_____

_____

_____

_____

What does Luke 2:51 say about how Jesus treated His earthly parents? Because we are called to follow His example, what does this mean for us?

_____

_____

_____

_____

_____

The Bible has much to say about honoring our parents. Look up each of the following verses and briefly summarize what it says about this issue.

Passage	What it says about this issue
Proverbs 20:20	
Proverbs 23:22	
Ephesians 6:1-3	
Colossians 3:20	
1 Timothy 5:8	

Some people are quick to say that we are only called to honor family members when they behave in honorable ways. Do you agree? Why or why not?

_____

_____

_____

_____

Reach out to someone in your family today. Speak or act in a way that honors him or her.

Dear God, may my words be kind and encouraging, uplifting and honoring those in my family, even if sometimes we don't see eye to eye. May I be a peacemaker in my family. Amen.

CHARACTER Day 3

When life squeezes, Lord, I'm afraid that all too often what comes out of me is impatience and frustration and worry. Please conform my character to Yours. Amen.

Some regard character as the person you are when no one is looking. Are you a person of kindness, integrity and good will? Or are you really just out for yourself? Honoring one another means displaying character traits that put others first. The notion of setting aside our own rights in order to fulfill our responsibilities toward others is almost foreign in today's culture. But it was also radical during biblical times. Read Philippians 2:5-11. Who is our supreme example of a person with a selfless character (see verse 5)?

_____

_____

_____

_____

What was Jesus' attitude about being God (see verse 6)?

_____

_____

_____

Even though Jesus is God, what four things did He do (see verses 7-8)?

1. _____

2. _____

3. _____

4. _____

What was the result of Christ humbling Himself in this way (see verses 9-11)?

_____

_____

_____

What character traits do you need to work on today in order to bring them in line with Christ's example?

_____

_____

_____

_____

What are some practical ways in which you will do this?

_____

_____

_____

_____

May I have the mind of Christ, dear Lord, and may I treat others in the way that Jesus would have me treat them. Amen.

ACCEPTANCE

Father, You accept me the way I am but love me too much to leave me there. May I, in turn, accept others where they are but also point them to You. Amen.

People feel honored when they feel accepted. Do you feel accepted in your First Place 4 Health group or in other groups at church? Why or why not? What about in groups outside of your church?

_____

_____

_____

_____

_____

What two reasons did Paul give to encourage us to "accept one another" (see Romans 15:7)?

1. _____
2. _____

Read James 2:1-13. What is James's warning in verse 1?

_____

_____

_____

_____

_____

What does James call the kind of preferential behavior described in verses 2-4?

_____

_____

_____

_____

According to verses 8-9, what sort of behaviors are right and what sort are wrong?

_____

_____

_____

_____

Have you ever been guilty of showing preferential treatment rather than accepting and honoring everyone as equal? How might you handle that situation differently now?

_____

_____

_____

_____

What specific words and actions make you feel accepted in a group? Which of these do you use to reach out in acceptance to others?

_____

_____

_____

_____

Father, sometimes I have looked askance at others who are different or seem to me to be somehow out of place. Help me to remember that all people are created in Your image and worthy of love and acceptance. Amen.

Day 5 AUTHORITY

Almighty God, You are the first authority in all areas of my life. But I know that I also must honor others in authority over me. Help me to do so in a way that honors You too. Amen.

We all live under authority. Americans are big on self-sufficiency, but the truth is we all answer to someone—usually several someones: boss, governor, parent, teacher, commanding officer, coach, minister—the list could go on and on. Read Daniel 7:13-14. What authority did Daniel see in his dream? What did this person look like?

_____

_____

_____

_____

Read Matthew 7:28-29. What did the crowds think about Jesus?

_____

_____

_____

According to Matthew 21:23, who actually questioned Jesus' authority?

_____

_____

_____

When Jesus finally described His source of authority, where did He say it came from (see Matthew 28:18)?

_____

_____

_____

_____

Who is the ultimate authority for Christians?

_____

_____

_____

According to Matthew 10:1, who was given supernatural authority and what were they to do with it?

_____

_____

_____

_____

_____

Read Romans 13:1-7. What does Paul say we are to do, and why (see verses 1-2)?

_____

_____

_____

_____

_____

What are two more reasons for submitting to authority (see verse 5)?

_____

_____

_____

_____

Even if we don't agree with the politics of an authority figure, what are we instructed to do (see verse 7)?

_____

_____

_____

_____

_____

While our ultimate authority is God Himself, we must also learn to treat earthly authority figures with honor and respect. When you agree with what authority figures are doing, it's pretty easy to honor them. But what about when you don't agree with them and what they're doing? What tools have you gained this week to better help you honor all authority figures?

_____

_____

_____

_____

_____

> *Lord, rather than be negative about all the abuse of authority I see in the world, please help me to show honor to those in authority so that I will have a positive effect on those around me. Amen.*

REFLECTION AND APPLICATION

Day 6

> *Heavenly Father, You continue to treat me as a precious jewel, yet I don't always treat as valuable others whom You created. Help me to see in them all the potential that You see in all of us. Amen.*

Most of us would agree that honoring someone means giving that someone special recognition, respect, compliments, the best seating, etc. When we honor someone, we show that we value that person. In 1 Corinthians 7:23, the word translated "price" is the same Greek word translated in other places as "honor." Its root word is usually translated "precious," "greater worth" or "dear." To honor one another, then, is to treat each person as precious, valuable or costly. Do you look at other people on the street as precious? Why or why not?

_____

_____

_____

_____

_____

C. S. Lewis once said the following about this idea:

> It is a serious thing to live in a society of possible gods and goddesses, to remember that the dullest and most uninteresting person you can talk to may one day be a creature which, if you saw it now, you would be strongly tempted to worship, or else a horror and a corruption such as you now meet, if at all, only in a nightmare. All day long we are, in some degree, helping each other to one or other of these destinations. It is in the light of these overwhelming possibilities, it is with the awe and the circumspection proper to them, that we should conduct all our dealings with one another, all friendships, all loves, all play, all politics. There are no *ordinary* people. You have never talked to a mere mortal. . . . But it is immortals whom we joke with, work with, marry, snub and exploit—immortal horrors or everlasting splendours. . . . And our charity must be a real and costly love, with deep feeling for the sins in spite of which we love the sinner—no mere tolerance or indulgence which parodies love as flippancy parodies merriment.[1]

How do our actions (or inactions) help a person to become a nightmarish horror?

How do our actions (or inactions) help a person to become a creature worthy of worship?

Dear Lord, You alone are the only creature worthy of worship, yet there are people all around me who could be more than they are if someone believed in them and urged them on. Help me to be that kind of someone. Amen.

REFLECTION AND APPLICATION

Day
7

Holy One, I have been learning so much about one-anothering through Your Word. Help me to not only recall it all but to put it into practice! Amen.

In the past weeks, we have examined many "one anothers" in the Bible, all of which are important. Take some time today to pray and think about each one, and note some of the lessons you have learned about each one.

Love one another

_____
_____
_____
_____
_____

Serve one another

_____
_____
_____
_____
_____

Be patient with one another

_____
_____
_____
_____
_____

Fellowship with one another

_____
_____
_____
_____
_____

Show compassion to one another

_____
_____
_____
_____
_____

Encourage one another

_____
_____
_____
_____
_____

Live in harmony with one another

_____
_____
_____
_____

Forgive one another

_____
_____
_____
_____
_____

Honor one another

_____

_____

_____

_____

_____

_____

O Jesus, grant me the grace to desire . . . that others may be chosen and I set aside . . . that others may be praised and I unnoticed . . . that others may be preferred to me in everything. O Jesus, grant me the grace to desire it. Amen.[2]

Notes

1. C. S. Lewis, *The Weight of Glory and Other Addresses* (New York: Harper Collins, 2001), pp. 45-46.
2. Merry Cardinal de Val, "Litany of Humility" (from the prayer book for Jesuits, 1963), *EWTN Global Catholic Network.* http://www.ewtn.com/devotionals/Litanies/humility.htm (accessed April 2, 2011).

Group Prayer Requests

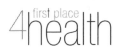

Today's Date: _____

Name	Request

Results

_____

_____

_____

_____

_____

_____

better together in godliness

SCRIPTURE MEMORY VERSE
*No one has ever seen God; but if we love one another,
God lives in us and his love is made complete in us.*
1 JOHN 4:12

During our *Better Together* study, we have looked at nine "one anothers" that are essential for our being better together. This week we will complete the study by emphasizing that the only way any of us can succeed in living out any of the "one anothers" is by God living in us and making His love complete in us. This is called godliness, and it is the lifestyle each of us should seek every single day. True godliness will not only help us live more balanced lives physically, spiritually, mentally and emotionally, but it will also ensure that we will indeed be better together.

Henri Nouwen has this to say about God's love:

> Jesus is the revelation of God's unending, unconditional love for us human beings. Everything that Jesus has done, said, and undergone is meant to show us that the love we most long for is given to us by God—not because we've deserved it, but because God is a God of love . . . Jesus . . . is God's most radical attempt to convince us that everything we long for is indeed given us. What [God] asks of us is to have faith in that love. . . . When Jesus talks about faith, he means first of all to trust unreservedly that you are loved [by God].[1]

The basis for our loving others comes out of the assurance that we are and will always be loved by God, our Creator. If we reflect on this truth and if we believe it with all our hearts, our lives will change forever.

Day 1

COMPLETION

Dear God, Your love is the basis for all that I am and all that I do. In other words, You are enough. Help me to know that Your love is what makes me complete. Amen.

Read 1 John 4:7-21, which is John's discussion of love. According to verse 7, why are we supposed to love each other?

_____

_____

_____

When we show love to each other, what two things do we reveal (see verse 7)?

1. _____

2. _____

How did God show His love for us, and why is that a definition of true love (see verses 9-10)?

_____

_____

_____

_____

What reason for loving others is found in verse 11?

_____

_____

_____

What did John mean when he wrote verse 12, this week's memory verse?

_____

_____

_____

Verses 13-15 further describe how God is able to dwell in His people. How does He do this?

_____

_____

_____

_____

According to verse 16, on what four truths can we rely, and why?

1. _____

2. _____

3. _____

4. _____

Why do we not have to be afraid (see verse 18)?

_____

_____

_____

According to verses 19-21, why can't we deny love to anyone?

_____

_____

_____

_____

*O Lord, I know that I can only love others because I am living in
the unconditional love that You so graciously give me. Your love
was sacrificial and has brought me life. I am eternally grateful. Amen.*

TRAINING

Heavenly Father, please deliver me from a life that never takes time for You. I want to grow in You. May I focus on all You have for me, and may I pursue You with gusto! Amen.

Seeking godliness is a daily discipline that is actually more about training than trying. In other words, we don't need to frantically strive to love one another; we simply have to commit to know God better, live out His Word and daily spend time in prayer and other spiritual disciplines so that His love overflows from our inner hearts. It really isn't that hard to do. In 1 Timothy 4:7, what are we told to do?

Read 1 Timothy 4:8. What is the reason for doing this?

Read 1 Corinthians 9:25. Why should we be like an athlete?

How is our prize different from that of an athlete?

What does a godly person do, and in what type of training does he or she take part? Why?

_____

_____

_____

_____

_____

Read 2 Timothy 3:16. What is particularly useful for training? Why?

_____

_____

_____

_____

_____

According to Hebrews 5:14, when we have been properly trained and are mature in our faith, what will be able to do?

_____

_____

_____

_____

_____

The term "spiritual disciplines" has the *D*-word in it —discipline! Any training for that which is truly important requires discipline. What are some ways you have had to exhibit discipline in each of these areas during this 12-week *Better Together* study?

Physical

_____

_____

_____

_____

Mental

_____

_____

_____

_____

Spiritual

_____

_____

_____

_____

Emotional

_____

_____

_____

_____

According to Titus 2:12, what does the godly person have to resist, and how are we called to live?

_____

_____

_____

_____

Remember that godliness and holiness should not be the focus of the Christian's life; they should be the fruit of a life wholly devoted to God. As our *Better Together* study draws to an end, how will you further train yourself to live a balanced life physically, spiritually, mentally and emotionally?

_____

_____

_____

_____

Dear Lord, You know it's hard for me to embrace training, but I have found true contentment through seeking You each day in an ordered way. Help me mature into godliness, step by step. Amen.

CONTENTMENT

Day **3**

O Lord, I want so much more—more of You and more time, more energy and more resources to serve You and others and really make a difference in the Kingdom. Help me be content with what You provide. Amen.

Think about someone you know who seems totally at ease with himself or herself, someone "comfortable in his or her own skin." According to Hebrews 13:5, how do we achieve this quality—this inner contentment—and why?

Read 1 Timothy 6:3-10. What are the characteristics of a person who is discontented (verses 4-5)?

What is the "great gain" that a contented and godly person gets (see verses 6-8)?

What happens to a person who is not content (see verses 9-10)?

_____

_____

_____

_____

Read Philippians 4:11-12. What does Paul say is the reason we should be content in any situation—good or bad?

_____

_____

_____

_____

Do you think that if you had a lot of money, a bigger house, more clothes—more stuff—that you would be happier; or do you think you would simply have different things to be discontent about? Why?

_____

_____

_____

_____

Read 1 Thessalonians 5:23. Are there any areas of discontent and strife in your life—anything that might prevent you from growing more like Jesus and being more godly? What prevents you from being content, and how can you change to become content?

_____

_____

_____

_____

Almighty God, I want to be content with my life as it is while I change to be more and more like You. I submit myself to You as You mold me into godliness and holiness, according to Your will. Amen.

EVERYTHING

*Dear God, my provider, truly You have given me everything I
need to live a godly and glorious life. Help me to become more godly
and to honor You with everything I do every day. Amen.*

Read 2 Peter 1:3-4. What one word describes what god has given us?
What is it that enables us to have this?

_____

_____

_____

_____

How do we avoid being corrupted by the world and what it thinks (see
verse 4)?

_____

_____

_____

_____

_____

How does a person get to know God better?

_____

_____

_____

_____

_____

What specific steps have you taken to get to know God better?

_____

_____

_____

_____

_____

Read Deuteronomy 6:5-6. What are we commanded to do?

_____

_____

_____

_____

_____

What will God do for those who obey these commands (see Deuteronomy 6:18)?

_____

_____

_____

_____

_____

Sometimes, we may fail miserably in our attempts to practice our "one anothers" and in our relationships. When this happens, we're liable to feel unworthy of God's "everything." We are not the first to feel this way. Read 1 Chronicles 29:14. Who else felt unworthy? Why did he feel this way?

_____

_____

_____

_____

_____

Read Mark 10:27. What is the difference between what is possible with a person's power and what is possible with God's power?

_____

_____

_____

_____

_____

Read Mark 9:23. What must you do in order to "harness" God's power for yourself?

_____
_____
_____
_____
_____
_____

Thank You, Father, for providing the power I need to achieve everything I need. Help me to always believe in You and Your promises. And thank You for never giving up on me, even when I falter. Amen.

FRUIT Day 5

Lord Jesus, truly You are the vine and I'm a branch that needs lots of pruning and watering and care. But I plan to stay close to You, and I deeply desire the fruit You will give through my obedience. Amen.

Paul prayed that the church at Philippi would be filled with what kind of fruit (see Philippians 1:11)?

_____
_____
_____
_____
_____

What actions result in this kind of fruit (see Philippians 1:9-10)?

_____
_____
_____
_____
_____

Read Psalm 1. What are the characteristics of each of the two types of people described?

Wicked	Righteous

According to Psalm 9:12-14, how long will the godly remain fruitful?

_____

_____

_____

_____

_____

Read John 15:1-5. Who is the gardener? Who is the vine? And who are the branches?

_____

_____

_____

_____

_____

What does the gardener do, and why (see verse 2)?

_____

_____

_____

_____

What are the branches to do in order to bear fruit (see verses 3-4)?

_____

_____

_____

_____

What happens if you are "apart from" Jesus, if you don't follow His commands (see verse 5)?

_____

_____

_____

_____

Are there areas in your life and in your relationships that you have been seeking to live "apart from Jesus"? If so, ask God to help you seek to live only through His power and presence and provision.

Father, sometimes I try to live apart from You, but You always draw me back. Thank You for daily nourishment and care. Amen.

REFLECTION AND APPLICATION

Day
6

Jesus, may I learn to love others well because You have loved me in a sacrificial and sanctifying way. May my love spill over to all around me. Amen.

What we think about is as important as what we do. In Philippians 4:8-9, we read the following:

> Whatever is true, whatever is worthy of reverence and is honorable and seemly, whatever is just, whatever is pure, whatever is lovely and lovable, whatever is kind and winsome and gracious, if there is any virtue and excellence, if there is anything worthy of praise, think on and weigh and take account of these things

[fix your minds on them]. Practice what you have learned and received and heard and seen in me, and model your way of living on it, and the God of peace (of untroubled, undisturbed well-being) will be with you (*AMP*).

According to these verses, how are we to live a godly and loving life?

_____

_____

_____

_____

What you think greatly influences what you do and what you say. Do you ever find your thoughts straying, and you begin to think about things that are bad for you or are flat-out wrong to think about? What can you do to get your thought-life back on a godly track so that you act and speak with love toward other people?

_____

_____

_____

_____

If we know and love God, the natural outcome will be to then love one another with that love given to us. As Catherine Hart Weber states:

> Loving others starts with our response to God's love. It is up to us to choose to reciprocate His love by loving Him back and then loving others. . . . Love as a mind-set, a daily way of being, becomes part of your intentional lifestyle, a habit and regular life practice. And it starts with a decision. When you learn to love imperfect people with God's unconditional love flowing through you, lives will change and you will change. If you will commit to do this, you will experience God's transforming love, which is filled with abundant, vibrant joy, peace, and hope.[2]

In what way(s) have you seen someone else's life changed by the love you have shown to him or her?

_____
_____
_____
_____

In what way(s) has your life changed because someone showed love to you?

_____
_____
_____
_____

In what way(s) has your life changed because of your love for God?

_____
_____
_____
_____

God, help me to always think, act and speak in a loving, godly manner; and help me reach out to others to let them know that You love them too. Amen.

REFLECTION AND APPLICATION

Day 7

Heavenly Father, will You transform me into a godly person who both receives and shows grace, mercy, love, hope, truth and gratitude every single day. Thank You for the gift of life and for the gift of life eternal. Amen.

As we receive God's love and we extend that love in us to others, we will be transformed. Read 2 Corinthians 3:18. Who will we begin to resemble?

_____
_____
_____

Author Frederica Mathewes-Green states the following about our transformation:

> God's presence in us is like the fire in the Burning Bush. It gradually takes us over, so that although we remain fully ourselves, we are being made over into our *true* selves, the way God originally intended us to be. He is Light, and we are filled with His light—maybe even literally, as some saints were said to visibly glow. The term for this transformation, is fairly scandalizing: *theosis,* which means being transformed into God. . . . Of course we do not become little mini-gods with our own universes. We never lose our identity, but we are filled with God like a sponge is filled with water.[3]

In Philippians 3:20-21, our obeying confirms that God will transform us. But why does Paul say that our citizenship is in heaven, not on earth?

_____

_____

_____

_____

_____

_____

_____

When we absorb God's love and allow it to transform us into His image, it's natural that His love in us will spill over into the lives of people around us. Our belief has earned us eternal life and, of course, we want others to experience the joy of living with God in heaven.

Take time today to really think about the sacrificial love that God has shown to you. Jesus died for you. Let that thought sink in. Then smile to yourself (and to God) because you know that you can live better for your own good and with others. We can be better together because we're better together with God.

Lord God, I pray that You bear lasting fruit in my life through the gift of the Spirit. You are the fountain of life. Enliven and refresh my listless, thirsting soul and spirit through Your love and vibrant life that renews. You are the tree of life. Make strong the branches of my life that have been weakened by the storms of daily life. Keep me fresh and filled with Your life. Your Spirit is living water. Deepen the roots of my restless and weary life through the river of life in Your Word. Refresh me and bring me joy by infusing me with Your Holy Spirit and more of Your abundant life. Your Church is the orchard that You feed and prune by Your love. Lord, I come to You longing for peace, nourishment, and to find rest in its shade. Amen.[4]

Notes

1. Henri J. M. Nouwen, *Letters to Marc About Jesus* (San Francisco, CA: Harper and Row Publishers, 1988).
2. Catherine Hart Weber, *Flourish: Discover the Daily Joy of Abundant, Vibrant Living* (Minneapolis, MN: Bethany House Publishers, 2010), pp. 110-111.
3. Frederica Mathewes-Green, "First Fruits of Prayer," quoted in Peter Scazzero, *Daily Office: Remembering God's Presence Throughout the Day* (Elmhurst, NY: Emotionally Healthy Spirituality, 2008), p. 33.
4. "Intercession," *Magnificat*, vol. 12, no. 5 (July 2010), p. 271.

Group Prayer Requests

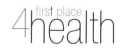

Today's Date: _____

Name	Request

Results

_____

_____

_____

_____

_____

_____

time to
celebrate!

To help shape your brief victory celebration testimony, work through the following questions in your prayer journal:

Day One: List some of the benefits you have gained by allowing the Lord to transform your life through this 12-week First Place 4 Health session. Be sure to list benefits you have received in the physical, mental, emotional and spiritual realms of your being.

Day Two: In what ways have you most significantly changed *mentally*? Have you seen a shift in the ways you think about yourself, food, your relationships or God? How has Scripture memory been a part of these shifts?

Day Three: In what ways have you most significantly changed *emotionally*? Have you begun to identify how your feelings influence your relationship to food and exercise? What are you doing to stay aware of your emotions, both positive and negative?

Day Four: In what ways have you most significantly changed *spiritually*? How has your relationship with God deepened? How has drawing closer to Him made a difference in the other three areas of your life?

Day Five: In what ways have you most significantly changed *physically*? Have you met or exceeded your weight/measurement goals? How has your health improved the past 12 weeks?

Day Six: Was there one person in your First Place 4 Health group who was particularly encouraging to you? How did their kindness make a difference in your First Place 4 Health journey?

Day Seven: Summarize the previous six questions into a one-page testimony, or "faith story," to share at your group's victory celebration.

May our gracious Lord bless and keep you as you continue to keep Him first in all things!

Better Together
leader discussion guide

For in-depth information, guidance and helpful tips about leading a successful First Place 4 Health group, study the *First Place 4 Health Leader's Guide*. In it, you will find valuable answers to most of your questions, as well as personal insights from many First Place 4 Health group leaders.

For the group meetings in this session, be sure to read and consider each week's discussion topics several days before the meeting—some questions and activities require supplies and/or planning to complete. Also, if you are leading a large group, plan to break into smaller groups for discussion and then come together as a large group to share your answers and responses. Make sure to appoint a capable leader for each small group so that discussions stay focused and on track (and be sure each group records their answers!).

week one: welcome to *better together*

During this first week, welcome the members to your group, provide a brief overview of the First Place 4 Health program, explain what is expected of the participants at each of the weekly meetings, and collect the Member Surveys. (See the *First Place 4 Health Leader's Guide* for a detailed outline of how to conduct the first week's meeting.)

week two: better together in love

In our memory verse this week, we are commanded to believe in Jesus Christ and love one another. Discuss which is the hardest of these two commandments to do and why.

Discuss some of the specific blessings that God promises to us in Leviticus 26:3-13 and John 15:10 when we obey Him. Ask the group where they most struggle with disobedience in the area of balanced health. How can naming this as they begin this study help them to be on the offensive? Ask those members who have already participated in a First Place 4 Health study what worked well for them in past sessions.

Ask the members to name some times when they tried to act in love toward someone but their heart really wasn't in it. Have them describe the results. Also have them think of a time when they continued to love someone even though it was hard. What were the results in that case?

Discuss some ways that the group members can "die daily" to their own will and their own way in order to show love for others. What does God consider us when we model Jesus' behavior?

We all start out well and plan to finish well, but sometimes life gets in the way and we fizzle. Ask the members what it will take for them to endure these next weeks toward balanced health.

Discuss some of the characteristics about love that the members recorded in Day 4. How is God's love different from the human love that we give and receive from others? What do we need to do to make our love more like God's?

Discuss how members of the Body of Christ should treat one another. Why are we commanded to love one another as "brothers"? Why is it often harder to act lovingly toward our own family than those with whom we are less familiar?

Conclude by asking the members to identify their primary love languages so that group can best know how to support them during this study. How do they expect to develop their love in each of the four areas of health—physical, spiritual, mental and emotional?

week three: better together in service

This week's memory verse encouraged the group members to use their gifts to serve others. What does this verse say about how they can administer God's grace to others? In what ways has God offered His grace to them by "stooping down" to lift them up?

In Day 1, the participants examined a list of gifts from Romans 12, 1 Corinthians 12 and Ephesians 4. Ask them to list the gifts that they discovered that God had given to them. How do they know that they have these particular gifts?

Talk about some of the ways we can exhibit humility as we serve others. According to the verses they studied during Day 2, what does God do for the humble? How does a humble person feel about others? How is this displayed in his or her life?

Discuss what it means to "serve others" according to the New Testament concept of the term (see Day 3). How have the members made themselves available and taken the time to pray through the prayer partner forms on a daily basis?

Have the group members give some of their thoughts on the story they read about Bishop Wellington Boone at the beginning of the Day 4 study. Talk about the main point that Jesus was trying to get across to His disciples by washing their feet. What are some ways that a person of even limited means could help to "labor" for God's kingdom?

Ask the members to list some of the acronyms they came up with that reflect their current behavior (see Day 5). One example might be ME: **M**yself first; **E**veryone else last. What is the dual meaning of the word *douleo* in the New Testament? How are we to exhibit caution in pursuing a healthy and balanced lifestyle for Christ?

In the sixteenth century, Saint Teresa of Avila said, "Christ has no body on earth but yours." Discuss whether this is still true 500 years later. If so, what can we do about it? When have the members been stretched to show kindness and compassion by serving others?

Conclude by asking the group members to consider how they can be more in tune with the voice of the Father so that they know when He is calling them to give up something in order to serve someone else.

week four: better together in patience

Discuss some of the times when the members have found it the hardest to be patient with others. Why is it that patience often doesn't come naturally to us? What are some of the actions of other people that try their patience the most?

The word "patience" is often translated as "long-suffering" in the Bible (see Day 1). What does James say about this in James 5:7-8? How does Paul say we are to exhibit patience in Ephesians 4:2?

Ask participants to name some instances where God taught them patience by giving them some sort of problem or affliction. How can hope and prayer help us to be more patient during difficulties? What is the result when we exhibit patience during the times of afflictions in our lives?

Discuss some of the words that come to mind when the members think of the word "meek." What was Christ's definition of this word (see Day 3)? What are the characteristics of the meek?

It's hard not to get upset when we see the wicked succeeding instead of the meek. Ask group members if they can think of a current situation in which they can test the words of Psalm 37 (see Day 3). What happens when we begin to worry about how better off everyone else seems to be than ourselves? What can they do today to start being more meek?

Discuss the differences between knowledge and wisdom and what makes a person truly wise. Have the participants briefly list some of the wisest people they know and what makes them so wise. Discuss the link between being patient and being wise (see Day 4).

Talk about some of the difficulties that Paul experienced during his ministry (see Day 5)? How do their difficulties compare with his? What kind of things are they steadfastly waiting on the Lord to deliver in their lives? What positive actions can they take while waiting for God's results/answers on their journey to a healthy and more balanced life?

Conclude by discussing why it is important to set time aside for God each day. Note that this was such an important command that God included it in the Ten Commandments (see Exodus 20:8). What did Jesus have to say about the Sabbath in Mark 2:27? How does a Sabbath day of rest restore a person and enable him or her to be a more patient person?

week five: better together in fellowship

Our fellowship with others tends to reflect what is going on within our own hearts. What did Jesus say about this in Luke 6:45? According to

Paul in Colossians 3:16, with what are we to fill ourselves? Given this, how can we prevent negative things from flowing out of us in our interactions with others?

Talk about why God calls us to live in fellowship rather than as "Lone Ranger" Christians. One way to do this is through hospitality. What is one thing about hospitality that they have learned from the Early Church (see Day 2)? According to Hebrews 13:2, why are we to treat others in a generous and cordial manner?

Ask the participants to list some of the ways they found in the psalms that we are to praise and worship God (see Day 3). Which of these ways were new to them? Are there any new ways that they would consider trying? If so, how will they incorporate that form into their worship?

One of the best benefits of life together in community is that we can support and encourage one another. This is where gathering together for instruction is beneficial. How have the members been supported and encouraged in their First Place 4 Health group? How has it helped them in instructing others? According to 2 Timothy 3:16-17, why is it so important to study the Word of God? How does it enable a person to recognize and reject false teachings both inside and outside the Church?

Discuss some of the ways in which we are called to exhibit a community spirit within our churches (see Day 5). How can we better exhibit a community spirit in our churches that models what occurred during the Early Church? How can we be a light to the world and *know* unbelievers without being *yoked* to unbelievers and allowing them to drag us down in our faith?

Conclude by discussing some of the ways the members believe God is calling them out of their comfort zone to experience community with those who are different from their normal circle of acquaintances.

week six: better together in compassion

Ask the members to review the letter from J. P. Kent in the introduction to this week's session. Why did the actions of the other inmates who gave up their items make such a strong impression on him? How did God use this situation to show love to him? Have they ever experienced compassion from strangers in a similar way?

Discuss the biblical definition of "mercy" (see Day 1). How does mercy differ from grace? What does it look like to extend mercy to others? According to Luke 6:36, why should we always do this?

One way we reach out with compassion is to offer comfort. Have the participants share a time when they were comforted and later were able to comfort someone else who was going through a similar experience. Why can we always count on God for comfort? How can studying the lives of other Christians who have been through trials similar to our own bring us comfort?

Discuss some of the ways in which justice goes hand in hand with compassion (see Day 3). Why is it often so hard to extend compassion to others who have wronged us? How are we following Christ's model when we do this?

Talk about some of the burdens we tend to carry around with us each day that weigh us down. According to 1 Peter 5:6-7, what are we to do with those burdens? What steps can we take to accomplish this? How can we help carry another person's burdens when our own are still so heavy?

Each of us is called to be a peacemaker. Discuss why peace is so important to fellowship and the difference between the peace Christ offers and the peace the world proposes. According to John 14:27, what does this peace that comes from Christ look like in a person's life?

Conclude by having the members review the second letter from J. P. Kent in Day 7. Ask them who has been "Jesus-with-skin-on" for them lately. How can such a simple gesture as giving a hug or opening a door for someone show compassion for others?

week seven: better together in encouragement

Ask the group members to describe who has been a "Son [or Daughter] of Encouragement" to them, just as Barnabas was to Paul. What is a phrase of encouragement that has helped them or that they have offered to someone else?

Discuss what it means to build each other up according to this week's memory verse (see Day 1). What does it mean to tear down another person? What are some tangible things they can do (or not do) to become more aware of places and times where others need encouragement?

In the Day 2 study, members read the following quote from C. S. Lewis: "Friendship is born at that moment when one person says to another: 'What! You too! I thought I was the only one.'" Ask them to give their reactions to this quote. In what ways has fellowship with other believers helped them to realize that they are not alone in experiencing particular problems?

Discuss why it is so important to be aware of what is really going on in each other's lives (see Day 3). How can we do this in love and be genuinely encouraging instead of overbearing? Why is it sometimes hard to be an encourager? Why is it so important to really listen to a person when he or she is talking instead of trying to formulate a solution to that person's issue in our mind?

Discuss what steps a person should take if he or she believes the Holy Spirit is prompting him or her to admonish another. Why is it important to pray and seek God first before we do this? What are ways we can prevent our admonishment from being misinterpreted by the other person?

Talk about why a person might be tempted to give up and stop seeking a life of balanced health and faith. How could that person be encouraged to persevere? According to James 1:2-4, what are we to do when we experience trials?

Conclude by asking the group members to state which memory verse in First Place 4 Health has encouraged them the most (see Day 7). Why has this verse been important in their lives? How has it helped them in a certain situation?

week eight: better together in harmony

When we seek harmony with others—even others quite different from ourselves—we become a pleasing and harmonious group. Discuss the four ways listed in 1 Peter 3:8 that can help us live in harmony with one another (see Day 1). What should we do in regard to people who are different from us (see Romans 12:16)?

Discuss the ways in which Paul compares the Body of Christ with the human body in Romans 12:3-21. Ask the members to consider what their role is in the Body of Christ? What is their role in their First Place 4 Health group? What reassurance can we gain from Scripture when we don't feel as if we belong (see Day 2)?

Talk about what happens when a watching world sees Christians at odds with one another. (Ask the members to provide some examples they have seen of this recently in the media.) What impression does this give to the world about Christians? How can they work to bring greater unity to your own community of believers?

On Day 4, the group members looked at unity and what it takes for each of us to bring unity into our own situations. Read Ephesians 4:3-6 and discuss what Paul states unites all Christians. Why is it important that this unity be maintained? In addition to glorifying God and bringing Him praise, what is another result of our unity in the eyes of a continually watching world?

Discuss what Paul meant in 1 Corinthians 3:1-4 when he said the believers were not ready for "solid food" (see Day 5). What was the cause of their setbacks? What was causing the division in the congregation? Why is it often difficult to avoid division in the Church?

Conclude by asking the members if they tend to accept the things they cannot change or if they tend to try to keep changing something (and, in the process, keep knocking their heads against a brick wall!). Where do they find the wisdom to know the difference between what they can and cannot change (see Day 7)?

week nine: better together in forgiveness

Read the quote from the introduction to this week's study: "Forgiveness is giving up your right to hurt someone back." Discuss why this can be so difficult to do.

Read John 31:13-15 aloud to the group. Ask the group what rationale Job used to choose to forgive others' grievances. Have they ever finally let go of a long-held grudge? If so, why did they hold on to it for so long? How did that grievance affect their relationships, and what happened when they let it go?

Discuss the biblical meaning of repentance from Day 2. According to 1 John 1:9, what two things happen when we confess our sins? What are some situations when they made a 180-degree turnaround in their lives?

Discuss the meaning of "redemption." According to Ephesians 1:7, what aspect of God's character offers us this redemption (see Day 3)? What is the result of our redemption?

Sometimes forgiveness is a process that takes time. Ask the group how God has been working out this process in their lives. How is He enabling them to forgive themselves for mistakes and bad choices they made in the past? How is He using them to help others not make the same mistakes?

Dr. Lewis Smedes said that when we forgive, "we set a prisoner free and discover that the prisoner is us." In what ways have the members seen this to be true in their lives? What does it mean to be a "slave to sin" (see Romans 6:7)?

Conclude by discussing some physical manifestations of spiritual misery and sin (see Day 6). Have the members review the list in Day 7 from Steven Curtis Chapman's facts about forgiveness. Which of these helped them to better understand what forgiveness *is* and *is not*?

week ten: better together in honor

The word "honor" can bring many images to our minds. Discuss with the participants what they picture when they think of this word. How are some ways that they typically show that they honor someone?

Discuss why it is often difficult to honor our parents and other members of our family. What commands do we find in the Bible telling us that we need to do this (see Day 2)? What benefits do we receive when we follow these commands? What can be the consequences if we don't follow these commands? Ask the members if they think they might find it easier to honor their family members after doing this week's study.

Have the members talk about some of their character traits that tend to seep out when no one else is looking. How can they begin to bring those under the lordship of Christ in a more godly way? In what ways will they follow Christ's example?

Discuss the two reasons Paul gives in Romans 15:7 as to why we are to accept one another (see Day 4). How can they show that they accept someone who is different from them? What specific words and actions make them feel accepted in a group?

Discuss in what ways Christians are called to live under authority on many different levels. When we do this in a practical way, how does it help our spiritual relationship with God? What are we instructed to do even if we disagree with the politics of an authority figure (see Romans 13:7)?

Ask the members to think about someone who is precious to them. Do they realize that God sees *them* that way? How can they encourage the godlikeness in others around them?

Conclude by discussing which of the nine "one anothers" they have studied thus far that have been the hardest for them to put into practice. Which has been the easiest? In which one have they improved the most?

week eleven: better together in godliness

Have the members review 1 John 4:7-21, which is the passage they studied in Day 1. According to John, how did God show His love for us? How should that affect how we love one another? How can God's love be made complete in those of us who are seeking to love one another? Can love and fear reside together in a person? Why or why not?

Seeking godliness is a daily discipline that requires training. Discuss what Paul tells us to do regarding this in 1 Timothy 4:8. According to Psalm 32:6, in what type of training does a godly person take part? What is the difference between training for godliness and striving to be godly?

Discuss some of the reasons why we should be content in any situation (see Philippians 4:11-12). Do "things" truly make a person happier?

If so, is this happiness short-lived or long-term? What prevents Christians from being more content? How can we begin to change that?

Talk about whether someone who is not grafted into the vine (Jesus) can bear fruit. Why or why not? According to Psalm 9:12-14, how long will the godly remain fruitful? What happens if we are "apart from" Jesus and don't follow His commands (see John 15:5)?

Conclude by discussing what is the natural overflow of a heart that is wholly committed to God, His will and His way. What are some of the fruit that is harvested in such a situation? What are some ways the group members can continue to seek godliness after this study ends?

week twelve: time to celebrate!

Even though most of your meeting this week will be a victory celebration, take some time at the beginning of the meeting to talk about how much God loves each person in the group and how each of us is called to love our brothers and sisters in Christ. (See "Planning a Victory Celebration" in the *First Place 4 Health Leader's Guide* for ideas about throwing a successful celebration for your group.)

For the rest of the study time, allow each member to tell his or her *Better Together* story. Give members an equal opportunity to share the goals they set for themselves at the beginning of the session and talk about the challenges and good things God has done for them throughout the process. Don't allow the more talkative group members to monopolize all the time. Even the quiet members need an opportunity to share their stories and successes! Even those who have not met their goals have still been part of the journey, so allow them to share and talk about why they did not succeed.

Making a commitment to continue in First Place 4 Health is an important part of victory. Be sure to talk about your group's future plans, and make each person feel welcome to continue to journey with you. One meaningful way to end your celebration would be to stand together in a circle and recite the *Better Together* memory verses. You could even hold hands with one another while you do it.

First Place 4 Health menu plans

Each menu plan is based on approximately 1,400 to 1,500 calories per day. All recipe and menu exchanges were determined using the Master-Cook software, a program that accesses a database containing more than 6,000 food items prepared using the United States Department of Agriculture (USDA) publications and information from food manufacturers. As with any nutritional program, MasterCook calculates the nutritional values of the recipes based on ingredients. Nutrition may vary due to how the food is prepared, where the food comes from, soil content, season, ripeness, processing and method of preparation. For these reasons, please use the recipes and menu plans as approximate guides. Consult a physician and/or a registered dietitian before starting a weight-loss program.

For those who need more calories, add the following to the 1,400-calorie plan:

- 1,800 calories: 2 ounce equivalent of meat, 3 ounce equivalent of bread, ½ cup vegetable serving, 1 tsp. fat

- 2,000 calories: 2 ounce equivalent of meat, 4 ounce equivalent of bread, ½ cup vegetable serving, 3 tsp. fat

- 2,200 calories: 2 ounce equivalent of meat, 5 ounce equivalent of bread, ½ cup vegetable serving, ½ cup fruit serving, 5 tsp. fat

- 2,400 calories: 2 ounce equivalent of meat, 6 ounce equivalent of bread, 1 cup vegetable serving, ½ cup fruit serving, 6 tsp. fat

First Week Grocery List

Produce

- ☐ angel hair slaw
- ☐ arugula, baby
- ☐ asparagus
- ☐ avocado
- ☐ bananas
- ☐ basil, fresh
- ☐ blackberries
- ☐ broccoli florets
- ☐ Brussels sprouts
- ☐ cantaloupe
- ☐ carrots, baby
- ☐ cauliflower florets
- ☐ cherry tomatoes
- ☐ chives, fresh
- ☐ cilantro, fresh
- ☐ cremini mushrooms
- ☐ cucumbers
- ☐ garlic
- ☐ ginger, fresh
- ☐ grapes
- ☐ green beans
- ☐ green onions
- ☐ lemon
- ☐ limes
- ☐ mint, fresh
- ☐ onion
- ☐ orange
- ☐ parsley, fresh
- ☐ pineapple
- ☐ plum tomatoes
- ☐ porcini mushrooms
- ☐ potatoes
- ☐ red bell pepper
- ☐ red onion
- ☐ red pepper
- ☐ romaine lettuce
- ☐ sage, fresh
- ☐ salad greens
- ☐ shallots, minced
- ☐ shiitake mushrooms
- ☐ spinach, baby
- ☐ sweet potatoes
- ☐ thyme, fresh
- ☐ tomatoes
- ☐ Vidalia onions
- ☐ watermelon

Baking/Cooking Products

- ☐ baking powder
- ☐ baking soda
- ☐ brown sugar
- ☐ canola oil
- ☐ flour, all-purpose
- ☐ honey
- ☐ molasses
- ☐ multigrain flatbread (such as Flatout®)
- ☐ nonstick cooking spray
- ☐ olive oil, extra-virgin
- ☐ sugar, granulated
- ☐ yeast
- ☐ yellow cornmeal

Spices

- ☐ black pepper
- ☐ chili powder
- ☐ cinnamon, ground
- ☐ cumin, ground
- ☐ nutmeg, ground
- ☐ oregano, dried
- ☐ salt

Nuts/Seeds

- ☐ almonds
- ☐ pecans

Condiments, Spreads and Sauces

- ☐ balsamic vinegar
- ☐ cider vinegar
- ☐ Dijon mustard
- ☐ Italian dressing, fat-free

- maple syrup
- mayonnaise, light
- pasta sauce
- mustard
- peanut butter
- picante sauce
- salsa
- soy sauce, low-sodium
- tomato paste
- white wine
- white wine vinegar

Breads, Cereals and Pasta
- acini di pepe
- bread, white
- brown rice
- chips, baked
- corn tortillas
- English muffins
- French bread
- Grape Nuts®
- panko, whole-wheat
- pizza crust dough
- sourdough bread
- spaghetti, whole-wheat
- tortilla chips, baked
- wild rice
- yellow rice

Canned Foods
- applesauce
- banana peppers, pickled
- black beans
- capers
- chickpeas
- corn
- ginger, crystallized
- green chiles
- jalapeño peppers
- navy beans
- pickles

Dairy Products
- butter
- buttermilk, fat-free
- cheddar cheese, reduced-fat
- Colby Jack cheese
- fontina cheese
- garlic-and-herbs spreadable cheese (such as Boursin light)
- half-and-half
- milk, fat-free
- milk, whole
- Monterey Jack cheese
- mozzarella cheese
- Parmigiano-Reggiano cheese
- ricotta cheese, part-skim
- sour cream, reduced-fat
- yogurt, fat-free

Juices
- apple juice
- lemon juice
- lime juice
- orange juice

Meat and Poultry
- bacon
- beef tenderloin steaks
- chicken breast, skinless and boneless
- chicken sausage with jalapeño peppers
- egg substitute
- eggs
- ground round
- ham slices, lower-salt
- pancetta
- pork tenderloin
- pork, ground
- salami
- salmon fillets, skinless
- shrimp
- tilapia fillets
- turkey breast slices, lower-salt

First Week Meals and Recipes

DAY 1

Breakfast

½ toasted English muffin topped with 1 tbsp. peanut butter and ½ banana
1 cup fat-free milk

Nutritional Information: 302 calories; 9g fat; 15g protein; 42g carbohydrate; 3g dietary fiber; 4mg cholesterol; 334 mg sodium.

Lunch

Chickpea Salad with Grilled Shrimp

¼ cup extra-virgin olive oil, divided
4 tsp. grated lemon rind, divided
¼ cup fresh lemon juice, divided
1 tbsp. fresh flat-leaf parsley, chopped
2½ tsp. crushed red pepper, divided
¾ tsp. salt, divided
½ tsp. black pepper, freshly ground
1 garlic clove, minced
18 large shrimp, peeled and deveined (about ¾ lb.)

6 cups canola oil
3 cups canned chickpeas (garbanzo beans), rinsed and drained
4 cups fresh baby arugula
2 cups fresh baby spinach
½ cup fresh mint, torn
⅓ cup fresh flat-leaf parsley leaves
⅓ cup green onions, diagonally cut (¼-inch)
nonstick cooking spray

Combine 1 tablespoon olive oil, 1½ teaspoons lemon rind, 1 tablespoon juice, chopped parsley, 1 teaspoon red pepper, ½ teaspoon salt, black pepper and garlic in a medium bowl. Add shrimp and toss well. Marinate in refrigerator for 1 hour, stirring occasionally. Clip a candy/fry thermometer onto the side of a Dutch oven. Add canola oil to pan and heat to 385° F. Dry chickpeas thoroughly in a single layer on paper towels. Place 1½ cups chickpeas in hot oil and fry for 4 minutes or until crisp, stirring occasionally. Make sure oil temperature remains at 385° F.

Remove peas from the pan using a slotted spoon and drain on paper towels. Keep warm. Return oil to 385° F and repeat the procedure with the remaining chickpeas. Remove shrimp from marinade, and then discard the marinade. Thread 3 shrimp onto each of 6 (5-inch) skewers. Preheat a grill to medium-high heat and place the shrimp on a grill rack coated with non-stick cooking spray. Grill shrimp for 2½ minutes on each side or until done. (You can also broil the shrimp skewers or cook them on the stovetop in a grill pan.) Combine the remaining olive oil, lemon rind, lemon juice, red pepper and salt in a large bowl and stir with a whisk. Add chickpeas, arugula, spinach, mint, parsley and onion and toss gently to combine. Divide the chickpea mixture between shallow bowls. Top each serving with 3 grilled shrimp. Serve with 6 wheat crackers and 1 cup diced pineapple. Serves 6.

Nutritional Information: 415 calories; 15.8g fat; 10.2g protein; 21.6g carbohydrate; 5.7g dietary fiber; 32mg cholesterol; 628mg sodium.

Dinner

Eggplant Parmesan

3 large eggs, divided and lightly beaten
1 tbsp. water
2 cups whole-wheat panko (Japanese breadcrumbs)
½ cup (2 oz.) fresh Parmigiano-Reggiano cheese, grated
2 (1-lb.) eggplants, peeled and cut crosswise into ½-inch-thick slices
½ cup fresh basil, torn

½ tsp. red pepper, crushed
1½ tsp. garlic, minced
½ tsp. salt, divided
1 (16-oz.) container part-skim ricotta cheese
1 (24-oz.) jar premium pasta sauce
8 oz. mozzarella cheese, thinly sliced
¾ cup (3 oz.) fontina cheese, finely grated
nonstick cooking spray

Preheat oven to 375° F. To make the eggplant, combine 2 eggs and 1 tablespoon water in a shallow dish. Combine panko and ¼ cup of the Parmigiano-Reggiano cheese in a second shallow dish. Dip eggplant into the egg mixture and dredge in panko mixture, pressing gently to adhere and shaking off excess. Place eggplant 1 inch apart on baking sheets coated with nonstick cooking spray and bake at 375° F for 30 minutes or until golden, turning once and rotating baking sheets after 15 minutes.

To make the filling, combine basil and ¼ cup Parmigiano-Reggiano cheese, red pepper, garlic, ¼ teaspoon salt, ricotta cheese and 1 egg. Spoon ½ cup pasta sauce in bottom of a 13″ x 9″ glass baking dish coated with nonstick cooking spray. Layer half of the eggplant slices over the pasta sauce and sprinkle eggplant with ⅛ teaspoon salt. Top with about ¾ cup of the pasta sauce. Spread half of the ricotta mixture over the sauce and top with

⅓ of the mozzarella slices and ¼ cup fontina. Repeat layers once, ending with about 1 cup pasta sauce. Cover tightly with aluminum foil coated with nonstick cooking spray and bake at 375° F for 35 minutes. Remove the foil, top with the remaining ⅓ of the mozzarella and ¼ cup fontina. Bake at 375° F for 10 minutes or until sauce is bubbly and cheese melts. Cool for 10 minutes and serve with a tossed green salad, fat-free Italian dressing and 1 oz. French bread. Serves 10.

Nutritional Information: 483 calories; 15.1g fat; 19.3g protein; 26.8g carbohydrate; 4.8g dietary fiber; 99mg cholesterol; 655mg sodium.

DAY 2

Breakfast

Sweet Potato Biscuits

2 cups all-purpose flour (about 9 oz.)
1 tbsp. granulated sugar
2 tsp. baking powder
5 tbsp. butter, chilled and cut into
   small pieces
½ tsp. salt
1 cup cooked sweet potatoes, pureed
   and cooled
⅓ cup fat-free milk
nonstick cooking spray

Preheat oven to 400° F. Lightly spoon flour into dry measuring cups and level with a knife. Combine flour, sugar, baking powder and salt in a bowl. Cut in butter with a pastry blender or 2 knives until the mixture resembles coarse meal. (Be sure to stop cutting in the butter while there are still pebble-sized pieces.) Combine sweet potato and milk in a small bowl and add potato mixture to flour mixture, stirring just until moist. Turn dough out onto a lightly floured surface and knead lightly 5 times. Roll dough to a ¾-inch thickness and cut with a 2-inch biscuit cutter into 10 biscuits. Place biscuits on a baking sheet coated with nonstick cooking spray. Gather remaining dough and roll to a ¾-inch thickness. Cut the dough with a 2-inch biscuit cutter into 6 biscuits and place these on the prepared baking sheet. Discard any remaining scraps. Bake at 400° F for 15 minutes or until lightly browned. Remove from pan and cool for 5 minutes on wire racks. Serve warm or at room temperature. Serve with 6 oz. fat-free yogurt and 1 cup blackberries. Serves 16.

Nutritional Information: 48 calories; 3.7g fat; 2.3g protein; 20.1g carbohydrate; 1.3g dietary fiber; 9.5mg cholesterol; 173mg sodium.

Lunch

Chicken Lettuce Wraps

2 tbsp. extra-virgin olive oil
2 tbsp. white wine vinegar
¼ tsp. salt
¼ tsp. black pepper
4 cups hearts of romaine lettuce, chopped
1½ cups skinless, boneless chicken breast, cooked and shredded

¾ cup (3 oz.) fresh mozzarella cheese, chopped
½ cup fresh basil, torn
1 pint cherry tomatoes, quartered
4 (2.8-oz.) pieces multigrain flatbread (such as Flatout®)
1 large garlic clove, halved
nonstick cooking spray

Combine olive oil, vinegar, salt and black pepper in a large bowl, stirring with a whisk. Add lettuce, chicken breast, mozzarella cheese, basil and cherry tomatoes, tossing to coat. Heat a large nonstick skillet over medium-high heat and coat pan with nonstick cooking spray. Working with 1 flatbread at a time, cook bread for 1 minute on each side or until toasted. Rub 1 side of each flatbread with cut sides of garlic. Arrange 1½ cups of the chicken mixture in the center of each flatbread and roll up. Serve with 1 ounce baked chips. Serves 4.

Nutritional Information: 468 calories; 15.9g fat; 30.3g protein; 22g carbohydrate; 9.5g dietary fiber; 61mg cholesterol; 573mg sodium.

Dinner

Salmon with Maple Lemon Glaze

2 tbsp. fresh lemon juice
2 tbsp. maple syrup
1 tbsp. cider vinegar
1 tbsp. canola oil

4 (6-oz.) salmon fillets, skinless
½ tsp. salt
¼ tsp. black pepper, freshly ground
nonstick cooking spray

Preheat broiler. Combine lemon juice, maple syrup, vinegar and canola oil in a large resealable plastic bag. Add fish to bag and seal. Refrigerate for 10 to 20 minutes, turning the bag once (do not marinade for more than 30 minutes). Remove the fish from the bag and place the marinade in a microwave-safe bowl. Microwave marinade on high for 1 minute. Heat a large ovenproof nonstick skillet over medium-high heat. Sprinkle fish evenly with salt and pepper. Coat skillet pan with nonstick cooking spray. Add fish to the skillet and cook for 3 minutes. Turn the fish over and brush marinade evenly over the fish. Broil for 3 minutes until the fish flakes easily when tested with a fork or until desired degree of doneness. Serve with ¾ cup wild rice and ¾ cup steamed asparagus. Serves 4.

Nutritional Information: 457 calories; 14g fat; 31g protein; 7.5g carbohydrate; 0.1g dietary fiber; 80mg cholesterol; 363mg sodium.

DAY 3

Breakfast

Gingerbread Waffles

2 cups all-purpose flour	2 tsp. peeled fresh ginger,
1½ tsp. baking powder	finely grated
½ tsp. baking soda	2 large egg yolks
¼ tsp. salt	1 (4-oz.) container applesauce
¼ tsp. ground cinnamon	3 tbsp. crystallized ginger, minced
1½ cups fat-free buttermilk	2 large egg whites
3 tbsp. canola oil	nonstick cooking spray
3 tbsp. molasses	

Lightly spoon flour into dry measuring cup and level with a knife. Combine flour, baking powder, baking soda, salt and cinnamon in a medium bowl and stir with a whisk. Combine buttermilk, canola oil, molasses, fresh ginger, egg yolks and applesauce in a small bowl. Add the milk mixture to the flour mixture, stirring just until combined. Stir in the crystallized ginger. Beat egg whites with a mixer at high speed until soft peaks form. Gently fold the egg whites into the batter. Coat a waffle iron with nonstick cooking spray and preheat. Spoon about ⅓ cup batter per 4-inch waffle onto a hot waffle iron, spreading batter evenly to edges. Cook for 5 minutes or until steaming stops and repeat the procedure with the remaining batter. Serve with 1 cup fat-free milk and ½ medium banana. Serves 9 (2 waffles each).

Nutritional Information: 353 calories; 6.1g fat; 5.8g protein; 32.5g carbohydrate; 1g dietary fiber; 47mg cholesterol; 277mg sodium.

Lunch

Grilled Ham and Turkey Sandwich

1 tbsp. light mayonnaise	8 (1-oz.) slices country white bread
1 tsp. Dijon mustard	4 (½-oz.) slices lower-salt ham

4 (1-oz.) slices lower-salt turkey breast

8 (¼-inch-thick) slices tomato

4 (½-oz.) slices reduced-fat cheddar cheese

nonstick cooking spray

Combine mayonnaise and mustard in a small bowl. Spread about 1 teaspoon of the mayonnaise mixture over 1 side of each of 4 bread slices. Top each slice with 1 turkey slice, 1 ham slice, 1 cheese slice and 2 tomato slices. Top with the remaining bread slices. Heat a large nonstick skillet over medium heat. Coat the pan with nonstick cooking spray. Add sandwiches to the pan and cook for 4 minutes or until lightly browned. Turn the sandwiches over and cook for 2 minutes or until the cheese melts. Serve with 15 baked tortilla chips and ½ cup salsa. Serves 4.

Nutritional Information: 412 calories; 5.8g fat; 18.4g protein; 29.1g carbohydrate; 0.4g dietary fiber; 28mg cholesterol; 781mg sodium.

....

Dinner

Glazed Pork Tenderloin and Carrots

¾ lb. baby carrots

¼ cup water

¼ cup honey

3 tbsp. apple juice or apple cider

2 tsp. Dijon mustard

1 tsp. low-sodium soy sauce

1 (1¼-lb.) pork tenderloin, trimmed

¼ tsp. salt

¼ tsp. pepper

1 tbsp. butter

2 tbsp. minced fresh chives (optional)

Place the carrots and ¼ cup water in a medium saucepan and bring to a boil over high heat. Reduce heat to simmer, stir, cover and let carrots simmer for another 10 to 12 minutes or until they are tender. Meanwhile, prepare the glaze by mixing honey, apple juice, Dijon mustard and soy sauce together in a small bowl. Set aside. When the carrots are done, remove from heat, drain and set aside.

Cut the pork tenderloin crosswise into 12 equal slices and season with salt and pepper. Melt butter in an extra-large nonstick skillet over medium-high heat. Add the pork and cook 2 to 3 minutes or until the pork is nicely browned on the bottom side. Using tongs, flip the pork over and cook another 3 to 4 minutes or until almost cooked through. Add the carrots to the pan with the pork. Stir the glaze again and add it to the pan. Bring the mixture to a simmer and cook until pork is done (about 1 to 2 minutes). Stir to coat pork and carrots with glaze. Divide the pork and carrots among 4 plates. Pour any remaining glaze over the pork and garnish with chives, if desired. Serve with ¾ cup brown rice and 1 cup salad greens with tomatoes and cucumbers and fat-free dressing. Serves 4.

Nutritional Information: 503 calories; 8g fat; 86mg cholesterol; 29g protein; 26g carbohydrate; 2g dietary fiber; 367mg sodium.

DAY 4

....

Breakfast

Sausage, Cheese and Egg Braid

1 (13.8-oz.) can pizza crust dough, refrigerated
1 tbsp. extra-virgin olive oil
¼ cup onion, chopped
4 oz. chicken sausage with jalapeño peppers, chopped
2 large eggs, lightly beaten

½ cup (2 oz.) Monterey Jack cheese, shredded
¼ cup reduced-fat cheddar cheese, shredded
¼ cup jalapeño peppers (optional), chopped and seeded
1 large egg white, lightly beaten
nonstick cooking spray

Preheat oven to 425° F. Unroll the dough onto a baking sheet coated with nonstick cooking spray and pat into a 15″ x 10″ rectangle. Heat oil in a large skillet over medium heat. Add onion and sausage and cook for 9 minutes or until lightly browned. Stir in eggs and cook for 1½ minutes or until set. Remove from the heat and sprinkle Monterey Jack cheese lengthwise down the center of dough, leaving about a 2½-inch border on each side. Spoon the egg mixture evenly over the cheese. Sprinkle cheddar over the egg mixture and top with jalapeño peppers. Using a sharp knife or kitchen shears, make 2-inch-long diagonal cuts about 1 inch apart on both sides of the dough to within ½ inch of the filling. Wrap the strips over the filling, alternating strips diagonally. Press the ends under to seal. Brush with egg white and bake at 425° F for 15 minutes or until golden brown. Let stand for 5 minutes. Cut crosswise into 6 slices and serve with 1 cup diced melon. Serves 6.

Nutritional Information: 217 calories; 10.4g fat; 10.6g protein; 7.3g carbohydrate; 0.1g dietary fiber; 98mg cholesterol; 344mg sodium.

Lunch

Taco Rice Salad

1 lb. ground round
1 garlic clove, minced
3 cups yellow rice, cooked
1½ tsp. ground cumin
2 tsp. chili powder
¼ tsp. salt
¼ tsp. black pepper
6 cups romaine lettuce (about
    10 oz.), torn
1 cup corn

3 cups tomato (about 1¼ lbs.),
    chopped
½ cup red onion, chopped
1 (15-oz.) can black beans, rinsed and
    drained
⅔ cup reduced-fat sour cream
⅔ cup picante sauce
½ cup (2 oz.) reduced-fat cheddar
    cheese, shredded
nonstick cooking spray

To prepare salad, heat a large nonstick skillet over medium-high heat. Coat skillet with nonstick cooking spray. Add beef and garlic and cook for 9 minutes or until browned, stirring to crumble. Drain and return the beef mixture to the pan. Stir in rice, 1 teaspoon cumin, 1 teaspoon chili powder, salt and pepper and cool slightly. Combine lettuce, tomato, corn, red onion and black beans in a large bowl and toss to combine. To prepare dressing, combine sour cream, picante sauce, 1 teaspoon chili powder and ½ teaspoon cumin, stirring with a whisk. Spoon dressing over the lettuce mixture and toss to coat. Place 1⅓ cups of the lettuce mixture on each of 6 plates. Top with ¾ cup rice mixture and about 1½ tablespoons cheese. Serve with 1 ounce baked tortilla chips and 1 cup watermelon. Serves 6.

Nutritional Information: 546 calories; 11.9g fat; 21.1g protein; 46.7g carbohydrate; 6.7g dietary fiber; 48mg cholesterol; 994mg sodium.

Dinner

Mushroom Bolognese

½ oz. porcini mushrooms, dried
1 cup boiling water
1 tbsp. extra-virgin olive oil
2½ cups onion, chopped
1 tbsp. plus ¾ tsp. salt, divided
½ tsp. black pepper, freshly ground
    and divided
½ lb. ground pork

8 cups cremini mushrooms (about
    1½ lbs.), finely chopped
1 tbsp. garlic, minced
2 tbsp. tomato paste
½ cup white wine
1 (14-oz.) can whole peeled tomatoes,
    undrained
¼ cup whole milk

10 oz. whole-wheat spaghetti,
uncooked
¼ cup fresh parsley, chopped

1½ oz. Parmigiano-Reggiano
cheese, grated

Combine porcini and boiling water in a bowl, cover and let stand for 20 minutes or until soft. Drain porcini in a colander lined with a paper towel over a bowl, reserving the liquid. Rinse and chop porcini. Heat olive oil in a Dutch oven over medium-high heat. Add onion, ½ teaspoon salt, ¼ teaspoon pepper and pork and cook for 10 minutes or until pork is browned, stirring to crumble. Add cremini mushrooms, garlic, ¼ teaspoon salt and ¼ teaspoon pepper. Cook for 15 minutes or until the liquid almost evaporates, stirring occasionally. Add porcini and cook for 1 minute. Add tomato paste and cook for 2 minutes, stirring constantly. Add reserved porcini liquid and wine and cook for 1 minute, scraping pan to loosen browned bits. Add tomatoes and bring to a boil. Reduce heat and simmer for 30 minutes, stirring occasionally (and breaking up tomatoes as necessary). Stir in milk and cook for 2 minutes. Cook pasta according to package directions, adding 1 tablespoon salt to the cooking water. Drain, toss pasta with sauce and top with cheese and parsley. Serve with tossed green salad with fat-free dressing and 1½ ounces of French bread. Serves 6 (serving size is ¾ cup sauce, about ¾ cup pasta, about 1 tablespoon cheese, and 2 teaspoons parsley).

Nutritional Information: 509 calories; 8.6g fat; 22.1g protein; 49.6g carbohydrate; 9.6g dietary fiber; 34mg cholesterol; 544mg sodium.

DAY 5

Breakfast

⅓ medium cantaloupe or
honeydew melon
1 cup fat-free yogurt

¼ cup Grape Nuts® cereal (sprinkled
on yogurt)

Nutritional Information: 281 calories; 1g fat; 15g protein; 57g carbohydrate; 5g dietary fiber; 3mg cholesterol; 345mg sodium.

Lunch

Monterey Jack Pasta Salad

6 oz. (about 1 cup) acini di pepe
(short tube-shaped macaroni)

2¼ cups plum tomato (about
14 oz.), diced

⅓ cup capers, rinsed and drained
¼ cup red onion, finely chopped
¼ cup pickled banana peppers, sliced
¼ cup fresh parsley, chopped
2 tbsp. cider vinegar
1 tbsp. extra-virgin olive oil
½ tsp. dried oregano

⅛ tsp. salt
2 oz. Monterey Jack cheese, cut into
  ¼-inch cubes
1 (16-oz.) can navy beans, rinsed and
  drained
1 oz. salami, chopped
1 garlic clove, minced

Cook pasta according to package directions, omitting salt and fat, and drain. Combine the remaining ingredients in a large bowl. Add pasta to the tomato mixture, tossing well to combine. Serve with 6 wheat crackers and a medium orange. Serves 4.

Nutritional Information: 512 calories; 11.6g fat; 16.6g protein; 51.7g carbohydrate; 6.3g dietary fiber; 21mg cholesterol; 919mg sodium.

....

Dinner

Almond-stuffed Chicken

⅓ cup light garlic-and-herbs spreadable cheese (such as Boursin light)
¼ cup slivered almonds, toasted,
  coarsely chopped and divided
3 tbsp. fresh parsley, chopped

½ tsp. salt
4 (6-oz.) skinless, boneless chicken
  breast halves
¼ tsp. black pepper, freshly ground
1½ tsp. butter

Toast the almonds in a skillet. Combine spreadable cheese, 3 tablespoons almonds and 2 tablespoons chopped fresh parsley in a small bowl. Set aside. Cut a horizontal slit through thickest portion of each breast half to form a pocket. Stuff 1½ tablespoons of the almond mixture into each pocket and secure each pocket with a wooden pick. Sprinkle chicken with salt and pepper. Heat butter in a large nonstick skillet over medium heat. Add chicken to the pan and cook for 6 minutes on each side or until done. Remove the chicken from the pan, cover and let stand 2 minutes. Top chicken with remaining 1 tablespoon almonds and remaining 1 tablespoon parsley. Serve with *Brussels Sprouts and Cauliflower Gratin* and 1 cup of steamed green beans. Serves 4.

Nutritional Information: 288 calories; 12.7g fat; 37.5g protein; 3.9g carbohydrate; 0.9g dietary fiber; 111mg cholesterol; 496mg sodium.

Brussels Sprouts and Cauliflower Gratin

4 cups Brussels sprouts (about 1¾
  lbs.), trimmed and quartered

4 cups cauliflower florets (1 lb.)
1½ cups fat-free milk

1.1 oz. all-purpose flour (about ¼ cup)
⅔ cup half-and-half
¾ tsp. salt
¼ tsp. black pepper, freshly ground
⅛ tsp. nutmeg, freshly ground
4 slices center-cut bacon, chopped

2 cups Vidalia (or other sweet onion), chopped
3 garlic cloves, minced
½ cup (2 oz.) grated Parmigiano-Reggiano cheese
¼ cup panko
nonstick cooking spray

Preheat oven to 375° F. Cook cauliflower and Brussels sprouts in boiling water for 2 minutes and drain. Lightly spoon flour into a dry measuring cup and level with a knife. Combine flour, milk, half-and-half, salt, black pepper and nutmeg in a bowl and stir well with a whisk. Set aside. Heat a large skillet over medium heat. Add bacon to the pan and cook for 3 minutes or until bacon begins to brown, stirring occasionally. Add onion and garlic and cook 5 minutes, stirring occasionally. Stir in milk mixture and bring to a simmer. Cook for 5 minutes or until thick, stirring constantly. Remove from the heat and stir in cauliflower and Brussels sprouts. Spoon vegetable mixture into an 7" x 11" broiler-safe ceramic baking dish coated with nonstick cooking spray. Cover the dish with foil coated with nonstick cooking spray. Bake at 375° F for 20 minutes or until bubbly, and then remove from the oven. Preheat broiler to high. Remove the foil from dish. Combine cheese and panko and sprinkle evenly over vegetables. Broil 5 inches from heat for 4 minutes or until browned. Let stand for 5 minutes before serving. Serves 8.

Nutritional Information: 148 calories; 5.2g fat; 8.7g protein; 18.3g carbohydrate; 3.8g dietary fiber; 17mg cholesterol; 399mg sodium.

DAY 6

Breakfast

Breakfast Burritos

1½ cups chopped tomato (about 1 large)
½ cup chopped green onions
½ cup chopped fresh cilantro
2 tsp. fresh lemon juice
¼ tsp. salt, divided
¼ tsp. black pepper, divided
dash of crushed red pepper

¼ tsp. chopped fresh oregano
4 eggs, lightly beaten
¼ cup chopped onion
1 (2-oz.) can diced green chiles
4 (6-inch) corn tortillas
½ cup (2 oz.) shredded Colby Jack cheese
nonstick cooking spray

To prepare the pico de gallo for the burritos, combine tomato, green onions, cilantro, lemon juice, ⅛ teaspoon salt, ⅛ teaspoon black pepper and a dash of crushed red pepper in a small bowl. To prepare the burritos, combine chopped fresh oregano, ⅛ teaspoon salt, ⅛ teaspoon black pepper, eggs and a dash of ground red pepper in a small bowl, stirring well with a whisk. Heat a large nonstick skillet over medium heat. Coat the pan with nonstick cooking spray. Add egg mixture, ¼ cup onion and green chiles to the pan. Cook for 3 minutes or until the eggs are set, stirring frequently. Remove the pan from the heat and stir the egg mixture well. Heat the corn tortillas according to package directions. Divide the egg mixture evenly among tortillas. Top each serving with 2 tablespoons shredded cheese and about ⅓ cup pico de gallo. Serve with 1 cup orange juice. Serves 4.

Nutritional Information: 307 calories; 10.8g fat; 12.7g protein; 14.3g carbohydrate; 2.4g dietary fiber; 258mg cholesterol; 372mg sodium.

Lunch

PLT Sandwich

2 tbsp. light mayonnaise
1 tbsp. shallots, minced
2 tsp. Dijon mustard
½ tsp. fresh sage, minced
2 oz. pancetta, cut into 8 thin slices

8 (1-oz.) slices rustic sourdough
  bread, toasted
4 medium tomatoes, each cut into 4
  (½-inch-thick) slices
1 cup baby arugula
nonstick cooking spray

Combine mayonnaise, shallots, Dijon mustard and sage in a bowl, stirring well. Preheat oven to 400° F. Arrange pancetta in a single layer on a baking sheet coated with nonstick cooking spray. Bake at 400° F for 8 minutes or until crisp and then drain on paper towels. Spread the mayonnaise mixture evenly over the bread slices. Top each of the 4 bread slices with 2 pancetta slices, 4 tomato slices and ¼ cup arugula. Top the sandwiches with remaining 4 bread slices. Serve with 1 cup grapes. Serves 4.

Nutritional Information: 392 calories; 8.7g fat; 10.5g protein; 41.9g carbohydrate; 3.5g dietary fiber; 13mg cholesterol; 699mg sodium.

Dinner

Beef Tenderloin Steak with Mushroom Sauce

4 (4-oz.) beef tenderloin steaks,
  trimmed (1 inch thick)

½ tsp. salt, divided
¼ tsp. black pepper, freshly ground

2 tsp. butter
2 garlic cloves, minced
4 cups shiitake or other mushroom caps (about 8 oz.), thinly sliced
½ tsp. fresh thyme, chopped

2 tbsp. balsamic vinegar
1 tbsp. water
1 tsp. low-sodium soy sauce
1 tbsp. fresh thyme leaves
nonstick cooking spray

Sprinkle steaks with ¼ teaspoon salt and ⅛ teaspoon pepper. Heat a large nonstick skillet over medium-high heat. Coat the pan with nonstick cooking spray. Add steaks to the pan and sauté for 3 minutes on each side or until desired degree of doneness. Transfer steaks to a serving platter. Heat a pan over medium-high heat. Add butter to the pan, swirling to coat, and cook for 15 seconds or until foam subsides. Add garlic to the pan and sauté for 30 seconds, stirring constantly. Add mushrooms, ½ teaspoon chopped thyme, remaining ¼ teaspoon salt, and remaining ⅛ teaspoon pepper to pan. Sauté for 3 minutes or until mushrooms are tender, stirring frequently. Stir in vinegar, 1 tablespoon water and soy sauce and cook for 1 minute or until liquid almost evaporates. Spoon the mushroom mixture over the steaks. Sprinkle with thyme leaves. Serve with 1 cup steamed broccoli and ½ cup mashed potatoes. Serves 4 (serving size: 1 steak and ¼ cup mushroom mixture).

Nutritional Information: 493 calories; 11.2g fat; 34.9g protein; 22.9g carbohydrate; 3.2g dietary fiber; 95mg cholesterol; 42mg sodium.

DAY 7

Breakfast

Pecan Sticky Rolls
¾ cup warm fat-free milk
¼ cup plus ⅔ cup granulated sugar
½ tsp. salt
1 package yeast (about 2¼ tsp.)
¼ cup warm water
½ cup egg substitute (or 1 egg)
7½ tbsp. butter, melted and divided

¾ cup packed dark brown sugar
18 oz. all-purpose flour (about 4 cups), divided
2 tbsp. hot water
⅓ cup finely chopped pecans, toasted
1 tbsp. ground cinnamon
nonstick cooking spray

To prepare dough, heat the milk to 100° F and then add in ¼ cup sugar and salt in a large bowl. Dissolve yeast in ¼ cup warm water in a small bowl and let stand for 5 minutes. Stir the yeast mixture into the milk mixture. Add egg substitute and 3 tablespoons melted butter and stir until well combined. Lightly spoon flour into dry measuring cup and level with a knife. Add 3¾ cups flour to the yeast mixture and stir until smooth. Turn the dough out onto a lightly floured surface and knead until smooth and elastic (about 8 minutes). Add enough of the remaining flour, 1 tablespoon at a time, to prevent the dough from sticking to your hands (the dough will feel slightly soft and tacky). Place the dough in a large bowl coated with nonstick cooking spray and turn to coat the top. Cover and let rise in a warm place (85° F) free from drafts for 45 minutes. Punch the dough down and turn over in bowl. Lightly coat with nonstick cooking spray, cover and let rise for another 45 minutes. Punch the dough down, cover and let rest for 5 minutes.

To prepare the glaze, combine brown sugar, 3 tablespoons melted butter, and 2 tablespoons hot water in a small bowl and stir with a whisk until smooth. Scrape the sugar mixture into a 9" x 13" baking pan coated with nonstick cooking spray, spreading evenly over bottom of pan with a spatula. Sprinkle the sugar mixture evenly with pecans and set aside.

To prepare the filling, combine ²/₃ cup granulated sugar and cinnamon in a small bowl. Turn the dough out onto a lightly floured surface and pat the dough into a 12" x 16" rectangle. Brush the surface of the dough with 1½ tablespoons melted butter. Sprinkle the sugar mixture evenly over the dough, leaving a ½-inch border. Beginning with the long side, roll up the dough in jellyroll fashion and pinch seam to seal (do not seal the ends of the roll). Cut the roll into 15 slices (approximately 1 inch wide). Arrange the slices, cut sides up, in the prepared pan. Coat the rolls with nonstick cooking spray, cover and let rise in a warm place (85° F), free from drafts for 30 minutes or until it has doubled in size. Preheat oven to 350° F. Uncover the rolls and bake at 350° F for 20 minutes or until lightly browned. Let stand for 1 minute and then carefully invert onto serving platter. Serve with ½ cup orange juice. Serves 15.

Nutritional Information: 330 calories; 7.6g fat; 4.9g protein; 47g carbohydrate; 1.4g dietary fiber; 15mg cholesterol; 146mg sodium.

....

Lunch
Sandwich and Salad

2 slices whole-grain bread
2 oz. cooked turkey or chicken
 breast, sliced

1 tsp reduced-fat mayonnaise
mustard, pickles and onions

Serve with tossed green salad mixed with sliced tomatoes, cucumbers, carrots peppers, 2 tbsp. fat free salad dressing and ¹/₃ cup pineapple tidbits. Serves 1.

Nutritional Information: 374 calories; 6g fat; 25g protein; 61g carbohydrate; 10g dietary fiber; 39mg cholesterol; 554mg sodium.

Dinner

Fish Tostadas with Roasted Corn Relish

½ cup reduced-fat sour cream
¼ cup salsa
1 cup corn
¼ cup red bell pepper, finely chopped
¼ cup red onion, finely chopped
1½ tsp. jalapeño peppers, minced
   and seeded
¾ tsp. salt, divided
1 cup avocado, peeled and diced
2 tsp. fresh lime juice

1½ lbs. tilapia fillets, cut into 2-inch
   pieces
¼ tsp. black pepper
⅓ cup yellow cornmeal
1 tbsp. canola oil, divided
8 (6-inch) corn tortillas
1 cup packaged angel hair slaw
lime wedges (optional)
nonstick cooking spray

Combine sour cream and salsa in a bowl. Heat a large nonstick skillet over medium-high heat. Coat pan with nonstick cooking spray and add corn, bell pepper, onion, jalapeño and ¼ teaspoon salt. Sauté for 5 minutes, stirring occasionally. Remove the mixture from pan and wipe the pan clean with paper towels. Combine avocado and juice and toss gently. Stir the avocado mixture into the corn mixture. Preheat a broiler. Sprinkle the fish evenly with the remaining ½ teaspoon salt and black pepper. Place the cornmeal in a shallow dish and dredge the fish in cornmeal. Heat 1½ teaspoons oil in a pan over medium-high heat. Add half of fish to pan and cook for 3 minutes. Carefully turn the fish over and cook for 2 minutes until the fish flakes easily when tested with a fork or until desired degree of doneness. Repeat the procedure with the remaining 1½ teaspoons oil and fish. Coat both sides of tortillas with nonstick cooking spray and arrange in a single layer on baking sheets. Broil for 2 minutes on each side or until crisp. Place 2 tortillas on each of 4 plates. Arrange 2 tablespoons slaw on each tortilla. Divide the fish evenly among tortillas and top each serving with about 3 tablespoons corn relish and about 1½ tablespoons sour cream mixture. Serve with lime wedges, if desired. Serves 4.

Nutritional Information:: 470 calories; 17.1g fat; 40.4g protein; 43.7g carbohydrate; 6.7g dietary fiber; 96mg cholesterol; 610mg sodium.

Second Week Grocery List

Produce
- ❑ apples
- ❑ asparagus
- ❑ bananas
- ❑ bay leaves
- ❑ blackberries
- ❑ button mushrooms
- ❑ cantaloupe
- ❑ carrots
- ❑ celery
- ❑ cherry tomatoes
- ❑ cilantro
- ❑ cucumbers
- ❑ dill
- ❑ fennel bulb
- ❑ fruit salad
- ❑ garlic
- ❑ ginger
- ❑ grapefruit
- ❑ green beans
- ❑ green bell peppers
- ❑ green onions
- ❑ green salad
- ❑ green-leaf lettuce leaves
- ❑ honeydew melon
- ❑ lemons
- ❑ mushrooms
- ❑ onions
- ❑ parsley
- ❑ peaches
- ❑ pineapple
- ❑ plum tomatoes
- ❑ potatoes
- ❑ radishes
- ❑ red bell pepper
- ❑ red onion
- ❑ romaine lettuce
- ❑ shallots
- ❑ sugar snap peas
- ❑ sweet potatoes
- ❑ tomatoes
- ❑ Vidalia onions
- ❑ watermelon
- ❑ yellow onions
- ❑ zucchini

Baking/Cooking Products
- ❑ brown sugar, light
- ❑ flour, all-purpose
- ❑ vegetable oil
- ❑ baking powder
- ❑ baking soda
- ❑ butter
- ❑ canola oil
- ❑ cornmeal
- ❑ cornstarch
- ❑ nonstick cooking spray
- ❑ sugar

Spices
- ❑ basil
- ❑ black pepper
- ❑ chili powder
- ❑ cinnamon
- ❑ cloves, ground
- ❑ cloves, minced
- ❑ cumin
- ❑ garlic powder
- ❑ oregano
- ❑ paprika
- ❑ red pepper
- ❑ salt

Nuts/Seeds
- ❑ cashews, dry-roasted
- ❑ walnuts

Condiments, Spreads and Sauces
- ❑ cider vinegar
- ❑ Dijon mustard

- [ ] honey
- [ ] ketchup
- [ ] margarine, light
- [ ] mayonnaise, light
- [ ] olive oil, extra-virgin
- [ ] red wine vinegar
- [ ] salad dressing, fat free
- [ ] salsa
- [ ] soy sauce, low sodium
- [ ] steak sauce, low sodium
- [ ] strawberry all-fruit spread
- [ ] Worcestershire sauce

Breads, Cereals and Pasta
- [ ] Arborio rice
- [ ] bagel
- [ ] bread, whole-grain
- [ ] bread stick
- [ ] cornbread
- [ ] couscous
- [ ] English muffins
- [ ] French bread
- [ ] Kaiser Rolls
- [ ] noodles, wide-egg
- [ ] pearl barley
- [ ] pitas, whole-wheat
- [ ] rice, long-grain rice
- [ ] spaghetti
- [ ] tortillas, flour
- [ ] wheat crackers
- [ ] wheat germ, honey-crunch
- [ ] wild rice

Canned Foods
- [ ] cannellini beans
- [ ] diced tomatoes
- [ ] navy beans
- [ ] beef broth, less sodium
- [ ] chicken broth, less sodium
- [ ] jalapeño peppers, pickled
- [ ] kalamata olives
- [ ] tomato puree, no salt added

- [ ] tomatoes, diced
- [ ] vegetable broth

Dairy Products
- [ ] cheddar cheese, reduced-fat
- [ ] cream cheese, 1/3-less-fat
- [ ] feta cheese
- [ ] milk, fat-free
- [ ] mozzarella cheese, part-skim
- [ ] Parmigiano-Reggiano cheese
- [ ] ricotta salata cheese
- [ ] whipping cream
- [ ] yogurt, fat-free
- [ ] yogurt, fat-free peach

Juices
- [ ] grapefruit juice
- [ ] lemon juice
- [ ] orange juice
- [ ] peach nectar

Frozen Foods
- [ ] hash brown potatoes
- [ ] mango pieces (such as Dole®)
- [ ] peaches, frozen
- [ ] peas
- [ ] whole-kernel corn

Meat and Poultry
- [ ] albacore tuna
- [ ] bacon, hickory-smoked
- [ ] chicken
- [ ] chicken breast
- [ ] chicken thighs
- [ ] chuck steak
- [ ] eggs
- [ ] ground sirloin
- [ ] ham, less-sodium
- [ ] lamb loin chops
- [ ] pork tenderloin
- [ ] shrimp, medium
- [ ] turkey Italian sausage

Second Week Meals and Recipes

DAY 1

....

Breakfast

Banana Muffins

⅔ cup light brown sugar, packed
¼ cup vegetable oil
1 large egg
1 large egg white
¾ cup ripe banana, mashed
⅓ cup fat-free milk

1⅓ cups all-purpose flour (6 oz.)
⅔ cup honey-crunch wheat germ
1½ tsp. baking powder
¼ tsp. baking soda
¼ tsp. salt
nonstick cooking spray

Preheat oven to 350° F. Combine brown sugar, vegetable oil, egg and egg white in a large bowl and beat with a mixer at medium speed until well blended. Add the banana and milk and beat well. Lightly spoon flour into dry measuring cups and level with a knife. Combine flour, wheat germ, baking powder, baking soda and salt in a medium bowl, stirring well with a whisk. Add to sugar mixture and beat just until moist. Spoon batter evenly into 12 muffin cups coated with nonstick cooking spray. Bake at 350° F for 22 minutes or until the muffins spring back when touched lightly in center. Cool the muffins in a pan for 5 minutes on a wire rack. Remove from pan and place the muffins on wire rack. Serve with 1 cup fresh blackberries. Serves 12.

Nutritional Information: 246 calories; 5.7g fat; 4.3g protein; 30g carbohydrate; 1.4g dietary fiber; 18mg cholesterol; 155mg sodium.

....

Lunch

BLT Salad

6 oz. French bread baguette, cut into
    ½-inch cubes
4 slices hickory-smoked bacon
1 tbsp. extra-virgin olive oil
¼ cup red wine vinegar
¼ tsp. black pepper, freshly ground
⅛ tsp. salt

6 cups romaine lettuce, torn
1½ lbs. plum tomatoes, cut into
    ½-inch wedges
3 green onions, thinly sliced
½ cup (2 oz.) feta cheese,
    crumbled
nonstick cooking spray

Preheat oven to 350° F. Layer the bread on a baking sheet and coat with nonstick cooking spray. Bake at 350° F for 18 minutes or until toasted. Cook bacon in a large nonstick skillet over medium heat until crisp. Remove the bacon from the pan, reserving 1 tablespoon of the drippings in a pan. Cut bacon into ½-inch pieces. Stir oil into the bacon drippings in the pan and remove from the heat. Stir in vinegar, pepper and salt to make vinaigrette. Combine lettuce, tomatoes, and onions in a large bowl and drizzle with vinaigrette. Add the bread and toss well to coat. Sprinkle with bacon and cheese. Serve with 2 slices fresh cantaloupe. Serves 4.

Nutritional Information: 362 calories; 14.4g fat; 10.5g protein; 37.6g carbohydrate; 4.7g dietary fiber; 26mg cholesterol; 788mg sodium.

....

Dinner

Pork and Vegetable Stir-fry with Cashew Rice

¾ cup long-grain rice, uncooked
⅓ cup green onions, chopped
¼ cup dry-roasted cashews, salted and coarsely chopped
⅔ cup fat-free, less-sodium chicken broth
2 tbsp. cornstarch, divided
3 tbsp. low-sodium soy sauce, divided
2 tbsp. honey
1 tbsp. canola oil, divided

1 (1-lb.) pork tenderloin, trimmed and cut into ½-inch cubes
2 cups sliced mushrooms (about 4 oz.)
1 cup chopped onion
1 tbsp. fresh ginger, grated and peeled
2 garlic cloves, minced
2 cups sugar snap peas, trimmed (about 6 oz.)
1 cup red bell pepper, chopped

Cook the rice according to package directions, omitting the salt and fat. Stir in ⅓ cup of the chopped green onions, chopped dry-roasted cashews and salt. Set aside and keep warm. Combine ⅔ cup chicken broth, 1 tablespoon cornstarch, 2 tablespoons low-sodium soy sauce and honey in a small bowl and set aside. Combine pork, the remaining 1 tablespoon cornstarch, and the remaining 1 tablespoon soy sauce in a bowl, tossing well to coat. Heat 2 teaspoons of oil in a large nonstick skillet over medium-high heat. Add the pork and sauté for 4 minutes or until browned. Remove from the pan. Add the remaining 1 teaspoon of oil to the pan. Add the mushrooms and 1 cup onion, and sauté for 2 minutes. Stir in the ginger and garlic and sauté for 30 seconds. Add the peas and bell peppers to the pan and sauté 1 minute. Stir in the pork and sauté for 1 minute. Add the reserved broth mixture to pan. Bring to a boil and cook for 1 minute or until thick, stirring constantly. Pour over cashew rice and serve with tossed green salad with fat free dressing and a 1 oz. bread stick. Serves 4.

Nutritional Information: 590 calories; 11.8g fat; 31.8g protein; 55.9g carbohydrate; 3.6g dietary fiber; 74mg cholesterol; 787mg sodium.

DAY 2

Breakfast

Peach Mango Smoothie

⅔ cup peaches, frozen and sliced
⅔ cup mango pieces (such as Dole®), frozen
⅔ cup peach nectar

1 tbsp. honey
1 (6-oz.) container organic peach fat-free yogurt

Place all ingredients in a blender and process for 2 minutes or until smooth. Serves 2.

Nutritional Information: 184 calories; 0.3g fat; 4.1g protein; 44g carbohydrate; 2.4g dietary fiber; 2mg cholesterol; 50mg sodium.

Lunch

Beef and Barley Soup

2 cups onion (about 1 large), chopped
1 lb. chuck steak, trimmed and cut into ½-inch cubes
1½ cups carrots (about 4), chopped and peeled
1 cup celery (about 4 stalks), chopped
5 garlic cloves, minced

1 cup pearl barley, uncooked
5 cups fat-free, less-sodium beef broth
2 cups water
½ cup no-salt-added tomato puree
½ tsp. salt
¼ tsp. black pepper, freshly ground
2 bay leaves
nonstick cooking spray

Heat a large Dutch oven over medium heat. Coat a pan with nonstick cooking spray. Add chopped onion and beef to pan and cook for 10 minutes or until onion is tender and beef is browned, stirring occasionally. Add chopped carrots and chopped celery to the pan and cook for 5 minutes, stirring occasionally. Stir in garlic and cook for 30 seconds. Stir in barley, beef broth, water, tomato puree, salt, pepper and bay leaves and bring to a boil. Cover, reduce heat and simmer for 40 minutes or until the barley is done and the vegetables are tender. Discard the bay leaves. Serve with a 2-ounce piece of cornbread and 1 cup pineapple. Serves 6.

Nutritional Information: 519 calories; 5g fat; 21.8g protein; 36g carbohydrate; 8g dietary fiber; 43mg cholesterol; 649mg sodium.

Dinner

Tomato Ricotta Spaghetti

2 pints cherry tomatoes, halved (about 4 cups)
5 tsp. extra-virgin olive oil, divided
½ tsp. salt, divided
8 oz. spaghetti, uncooked

⅓ cup fresh basil, chopped
¼ tsp. black pepper, freshly ground
½ cup (2 oz.) ricotta salata cheese, crumbled

Preheat oven to 400° F. Place tomatoes on a foil-lined baking sheet. Drizzle with 1 teaspoon oil and sprinkle with ⅛ teaspoon salt. Bake at 400° F for 20 minutes or until the tomatoes collapse. Cook the pasta according to package directions, omitting salt and fat. Drain the pasta in a colander over a bowl, reserving ⅓ cup of the cooking liquid. Return the pasta and reserved liquid to pan and stir in tomatoes, remaining 4 teaspoons oil, remaining ⅜ teaspoon salt, basil, pepper and cheese. Toss well. Serve with a tossed green salad with fat-free dressing and a 1½ oz. piece of French bread. Serves 4.

Nutritional Information: 314 calories; 8.4g fat; 10.5g protein; 50.3g carbohydrate; 3.6g dietary fiber; 4.6mg cholesterol; 331mg sodium.

DAY 3

Breakfast

1 (2 oz.) English muffin
1 tsp. light margarine
½ medium grapefruit

1 cup fat-free milk

Nutritional Information: 273 calories; 3g fat; 13g protein; 48g carbohydrate; 3g dietary fiber; 4mg cholesterol; 435mg sodium.

Lunch

Vegetable Soup with Corn Dumplings

1 tbsp. extra-virgin olive oil
4 cups onion, finely chopped
⅛ tsp. cloves, ground
4 garlic cloves, minced
2 bay leaves
3 cups water
3 (14½-oz.) cans vegetable broth
1 (14½-oz.) can diced tomatoes, undrained
1½ cups sweet potato, peeled and diced
1 (15-oz.) can navy beans, rinsed and drained
2⅓ cups frozen whole-kernel corn, divided
2 cups zucchini, sliced
¼ cup fresh parsley, chopped
⅛ tsp. ground red pepper
¾ cup all-purpose flour
1 tbsp. cornmeal
1½ tsp. baking powder
1 tsp. sugar
½ tsp. salt
1 tbsp. butter
½ cup fat-free milk

To prepare soup, heat olive oil in a large Dutch oven over medium heat. Add onion, cloves, garlic and bay leaves and cook for 10 minutes. Add water, broth and tomatoes and bring to a boil. Add sweet potato and beans and cook for 10 minutes. Stir in 2 cups corn, zucchini, parsley and red pepper and bring to a boil. Reduce heat and simmer for 5 minutes. Discard bay leaves. To prepare dumplings, combine flour, cornmeal, baking powder, sugar and salt in a bowl. Cut in butter with a pastry blender or 2 knives until the mixture resembles coarse meal. Add the milk and ⅓ cup corn and stir just until moist. Bring the soup to a boil. Drop the dumpling dough by rounded tablespoonfuls into the vegetable mixture to form 8 dumplings. Cover, reduce heat and cook over medium-low heat for 10 minutes or until the dumplings are done (do not boil). Serve with 1 medium sliced apple added to ½ cup of grapes. Serves 8.

Nutritional Information: 398 calories; 4.9g fat; 11g protein; 50.9g carbohydrate; 7.5g dietary fiber; 4mg cholesterol; 767mg sodium.

Dinner

Spicy Honey Chicken Thighs

2 tsp. garlic powder
2 tsp. chili powder
¾ tsp. salt
1 tsp. ground cumin
1 tsp. paprika
½ tsp. ground red pepper
8 skinless, boneless chicken thighs
6 tbsp. honey
2 tsp. cider vinegar
nonstick cooking spray

Preheat broiler. Combine garlic powder, chili powder, salt, cumin, paprika and red pepper in a large bowl. Add chicken to the bowl and toss to coat. Place the chicken on a broiler pan coated with nonstick cooking spray. Broil the chicken 5 minutes on each side. Combine the honey and vinegar in a small bowl, stirring well. Remove the chicken from the oven and brush ¼ cup of the honey mixture over it. Broil for 1 minute. Remove the chicken from oven and turn over. Brush the chicken with the remaining honey mixture. Broil for 1 additional minute or until the chicken is done. Serve with ¾ cup wild rice and 1 cup steamed green beans. Serves 4.

Nutritional Information: 515 calories; 11g fat; 28g protein; 27.9g carbohydrate; 0.6g dietary fiber; 99mg cholesterol; 528mg sodium.

DAY 4

Breakfast

Lumberjack Hash

2 tsp. vegetable oil	8 cups frozen hash brown potatoes,
2 tsp. butter	thawed (about 1 lb.)
1 cup onion, chopped	½ tsp. black pepper
1 cup green bell pepper, chopped	4 oz. less-sodium ham, diced
2 garlic cloves, minced	¾ cup (3 oz.) reduced-fat cheddar
½ tsp. salt	cheese, shredded

Heat the oil and butter in a large nonstick skillet over medium heat. Add onion and cook for 5 minutes. Add bell pepper and garlic and cook for 3 minutes. Add potatoes, salt, pepper and ham and cook for 16 minutes or until the potatoes are golden brown, stirring occasionally. Top with cheese and cook for 2 minutes or until the cheese melts. Serve with ½ cup orange or grapefruit juice. Serves 4.

Nutritional Information: 331 calories; 9.1g fat; 16.5g protein; 33.7g carbohydrate; 3.5g dietary fiber; 33mg cholesterol; 738mg sodium.

Lunch

Chicken, Cucumber and Carrot Salad

2 cups chicken breast (about 1 lb.), cooked and chopped	1¼ cups seeded cucumber, chopped
	½ cup carrots, matchstick-cut

½ cup radishes, sliced
⅓ cup green onions, chopped
¼ cup light mayonnaise
2 tbsp. fresh cilantro, chopped
1 tsp. garlic, minced
¼ tsp. salt

¼ tsp. ground cumin
⅛ tsp. black pepper
4 green-leaf lettuce leaves
4 (6-inch) whole-wheat pitas,
    cut into 8 wedges

Combine chicken breast, cucumber, carrots, radishes and onions in a large bowl. Combine mayonnaise, cilantro, garlic, salt, cumin and pepper in a small bowl, stirring with a whisk. Add the mayonnaise mixture to the chicken mixture and stir until combined. Place 1 lettuce leaf on each of 4 plates and top each leaf with about 1 cup of the chicken mixture. Place 8 pita wedges on each serving. Serve with a medium sliced peach. Serves 4.

Nutritional Information: 420 calories; 10.4g fat; 40.7g protein; 31.4g carbohydrate; 5.1g dietary fiber; 102mg cholesterol; 621mg sodium.

....

Dinner

Shrimp and Asparagus Risotto

3 cups fat-free, less-sodium chicken
    broth
1 cup water
2 tsp. extra-virgin olive oil
2¾ cups Vidalia or other sweet onion
    (about 2 medium), chopped
1 cup Arborio rice
2 garlic cloves, minced

1¾ cups (½-inch pieces) asparagus
1 lb. medium shrimp, peeled and
    deveined and cut into 1-inch pieces
½ cup (2 oz.) feta cheese, crumbled
1 tbsp. fresh dill, chopped
2 tbsp. fresh lemon juice
¼ tsp. salt
⅛ tsp. black pepper, freshly ground

Bring broth and water to a simmer in a medium saucepan (do not boil). Keep warm over low heat. Heat oil in a large saucepan over medium-high heat. Add onion to the pan and sauté for 5 minutes or until tender. Stir in rice and garlic and sauté for 1 minute. Add the broth mixture, ½ cup at a time, stirring constantly until each portion of the broth is absorbed before adding the next (about 30 minutes total). Stir in asparagus and shrimp and cook for 5 minutes or until the shrimp are done, stirring constantly. Remove from heat and stir in cheese, dill, lemon juice, salt and pepper. Serve with tossed green salad and fat-free dressing. Serves 4.

Nutritional Information: 476 calories; 8.9g fat; 33g protein; 53.5g carbohydrate; 5.1g dietary fiber; 189mg cholesterol; 868mg sodium.

DAY 5

Breakfast

Bagel and Berries

1 small (2 oz.) bagel
1 tsp. strawberry all-fruit spread
¾ cup fat-free yogurt
¾ cup blackberries

Nutritional Information: 318 calories; 2g fat; 14g protein; 64g carbohydrate; 9g dietary fiber; 2mg cholesterol; 401mg sodium.

Lunch

French Bread Pizza

1½ cups onion, vertically sliced
1 cup green bell pepper, cut into strips
2 (4-oz.) links turkey Italian sausage
¼ tsp. red pepper, crushed
1 (14.5-oz.) can diced tomatoes, undrained
1 (8-oz.) loaf French bread, cut in half horizontally
1 cup (4 oz.) part-skim mozzarella cheese, shredded
nonstick cooking spray

Preheat oven to 450° F. Heat a large nonstick skillet coated with nonstick cooking spray over medium-high heat. Add sliced onion and green bell pepper strips and sauté for 6 minutes or until tender. Remove casings from the sausage. Add the sausage to the pan and cook for 5 minutes or until lightly browned, stirring to crumble. Add crushed red pepper and diced tomatoes and cook for 5 minutes or until mixture thickens. Spread the sausage mixture evenly over cut sides of bread and sprinkle evenly with cheese. Place the bread halves on a baking sheet. Bake at 450° F for 5 minutes or until the cheese melts. Cut each pizza in half. Serve with a medium apple. Serves 4.

Nutritional Information: 447 calories; 12g fat; 24.6g protein; 42g carbohydrate; 4.9g dietary fiber; 63mg cholesterol; 967mg sodium.

Dinner

Smothered Steak Burgers

2 tbsp. shallots, finely chopped
1 garlic clove, minced
1 (8-oz.) package pre-sliced button mushrooms
½ cup fat-free, less-sodium beef broth
1 tbsp. low-sodium steak sauce
1 tsp. cornstarch

½ tsp. black pepper, freshly ground
and divided
2 tbsp. ketchup
1 tbsp. Worcestershire sauce
1 lb. ground sirloin

¼ tsp. salt
4 green-leaf lettuce leaves
4 (½-inch-thick) tomato slices
4 (2-oz.) Kaiser Rolls, toasted
nonstick cooking spray

Heat a large nonstick skillet over medium heat. Coat the pan with nonstick cooking spray. Add shallots and garlic to the pan and cook for 1 minute or until tender, stirring frequently. Increase heat to medium-high. Add mushrooms to the pan and cook for 10 minutes or until the moisture evaporates, stirring occasionally. Combine broth, steak sauce and cornstarch, stirring with a whisk. Add the broth mixture to the pan and bring to a boil. Cook for 1 minute or until thickened, stirring constantly. Stir in ¼ teaspoon pepper. Remove the mushroom mixture from pan, cover and keep warm. Wipe the pan with paper towels. Combine the remaining ¼ teaspoon pepper, ketchup and Worcestershire sauce in a large bowl, stirring with a whisk. Add beef to the bowl and toss gently to combine. Shape the beef mixture into 4 (½-inch-thick) patties and sprinkle evenly with salt. Heat a pan over medium-high heat. Coat the pan with nonstick cooking spray. Add patties to the pan and cook for 4 minutes. Turn and cook for 3 minutes or until desired degree of doneness. Place 1 lettuce leaf and 1 tomato slice on the bottom half of each roll. Top each serving with 1 patty, about ¼ cup of the mushroom mixture, and the top half of each roll. Serve with ¾ cup roasted potato wedges and 1 cup watermelon. Serves 4.

Nutritional Information: 519 calories; 12.9g fat; 30.7g protein; 38.4g carbohydrate; 1.9g dietary fiber; 41mg cholesterol; 747mg sodium.

DAY 6

Breakfast

Baked Eggs
1 tbsp. butter
6 large eggs
1 tsp. black pepper, freshly ground

¾ tsp. salt
2 tbsp. whipping cream

Preheat oven to 350° F. Coat each of 6 (6-ounce) ramekins or custard cups with ½ teaspoon butter. Break 1 egg into each prepared ramekin. Sprinkle eggs evenly with pepper and salt and spoon 1 teaspoon of the whipping cream over each egg. Place ramekins in a 9″ x 13″ baking dish and add hot water to pan to a depth of 1¼ inches. Bake at 350° F for 25 minutes or until the eggs are set. Serve with 1 cup orange juice and 1 piece light wholegrain toast with 1 teaspoon butter. Serves 6.

Nutritional Information: 292 calories; 8.7g fat; 6.5g protein; 0.8g carbohydrate; 0.1g dietary fiber; 223mg cholesterol; 380mg sodium.

Lunch

Mediterranean Barley Salad

2¼ cups water
¾ cup pearl barley, uncooked
1½ tsp. lemon rind, grated
3 tbsp. fresh lemon juice
2 tbsp. extra-virgin olive oil
½ tsp. Dijon mustard
1 cup fennel bulb, thinly sliced
⅓ cup fresh parsley, chopped
¼ cup red onion, finely chopped
¾ tsp. salt
½ tsp. black pepper, coarsely ground
8 pitted kalamata olives, halved
1 (15-oz.) can cannellini beans, rinsed and drained
⅓ cup walnuts, chopped and toasted

Bring water and barley to a boil in a saucepan. Cover, reduce heat and simmer for 25 minutes or until tender and the liquid is almost absorbed. Cool to room temperature. Combine lemon rind, lemon juice, olive oil and mustard in a bowl and stir well with a whisk. Add barley, fennel, parsley, red onion, salt, pepper, olives, and cannellini beans and toss gently. Cover and refrigerate for 30 minutes. Garnish with walnuts just before serving. Serve with 6 wheat crackers. Serves 4.

Nutritional Information: 392 calories; 16.1g fat; 6.6g protein; 38.9g carbohydrate; 8.2g dietary fiber; 0.0mg cholesterol; 643mg sodium.

Dinner

Tuna Noodle Casserole

8 oz. wide-egg noodles
2 tbsp. extra-virgin olive oil
½ cup yellow onion, chopped
⅓ cup carrot, chopped
2 tbsp. all-purpose flour
2¾ cups fat-free milk
2 tbsp. Dijon mustard
½ cup (4 oz.) ⅓-less-fat cream cheese, softened
¼ tsp. salt
½ tsp. black pepper, freshly ground
1 cup frozen peas, thawed
½ cup (2 oz.) Parmigiano-Reggiano cheese, grated and divided
2 (5-oz.) cans albacore tuna in water, drained and flaked
nonstick cooking spray

Preheat broiler. Cook noodles according to package directions, omitting salt and fat, and drain. Heat a large skillet over medium heat. Add oil to the pan and swirl to coat. Add onion and carrot and cook for 6 minutes or until carrot is almost tender, stirring occasionally. Sprinkle with flour and cook for 1 minute, stirring constantly. Gradually stir in milk and cook 5 minutes, stirring constantly with a whisk until slightly thick. Stir in cream cheese, mustard, salt and pepper and cook for 2 minutes, stirring constantly. Remove pan from the heat. Stir in noodles, peas, ¼ cup Parmigiano-Reggiano cheese and tuna. Spoon the mixture into a shallow broiler-safe 2-quart baking dish coated with nonstick cooking spray. Top with the remaining ¼ cup Parmigiano-Reggiano cheese. Broil for 3 minutes or until golden and bubbly. Let stand for 5 minutes before serving. Serve with 1 cup fresh fruit salad. Serves 6.

Nutritional Information: 487 calories; 16.5g fat; 27.4g protein; 40.6g carbohydrate; 3g dietary fiber; 88mg cholesterol; 608mg sodium.

DAY 7

Breakfast

Toast with Cinnamon

1 slice whole-grain bread, toasted   ½ tsp sugar
1 tsp. light margarine   pinch of cinnamon

Top bread with margarine, sugar and cinnamon. Serve with 6 ounces non-fat yogurt and ¾ cup berries. Serves 1.

Nutritional Information: 319 calories; 5g fat; 16g protein; 56g carbohydrate; 7g dietary fiber; 3mg cholesterol; 478mg sodium.

Lunch

Spicy Chicken Quesadillas

¼ cup green onions, thinly sliced   4 (8-inch) flour tortillas
2 tbsp. cilantro, chopped   ¾ cup (3 oz.) reduced-fat shredded
1 tbsp. pickled jalapeño peppers   cheddar cheese, divided
1 cup chicken (about 8 oz.), chopped,   ¾ cup salsa
   cooked and divided   nonstick cooking spray

Combine green onions, cilantro and jalapeño peppers in a small bowl and stir until blended. Place ¼ cup chopped chicken over half of 1 tortilla. Sprinkle with 3 tablespoons cheese and 1 tablespoon of the onion mixture and fold in half. Repeat procedure with the remaining tortillas, chicken, cheese and onion mixture. Heat a large nonstick skillet over medium-high heat. Coat pan with nonstick cooking spray. Place 2 quesadillas in the pan. Cook for 2 minutes on each side or until lightly browned. Repeat procedure with remaining quesadillas. Cut each quesadilla in half and serve with salsa. Serve with 1 cup honeydew melon. Serves 4.

Nutritional Information: 389 calories; 10.9g fat; 27.9g protein; 29.4g carbohydrate; 2.1g dietary fiber; 65mg cholesterol; 786mg sodium.

Dinner

Lamb Chops with Olive Couscous

1 tbsp. dried oregano
2 tbsp. extra-virgin olive oil
½ tsp. black pepper
3 garlic cloves, minced
8 (4-oz.) lamb loin chops, trimmed
½ tsp. salt
1 cup couscous, uncooked

1 (14-oz.) can fat-free, less-sodium chicken broth
½ cup cherry tomatoes, halved
¼ cup kalamata olives, pitted and chopped
3 tbsp. feta cheese, crumbled
nonstick cooking spray

Preheat broiler. Combine oregano, olive oil, pepper and cloves in a bowl. Sprinkle the lamb with salt and rub with 1 tablespoon of the oil mixture. Place on a broiler pan coated with nonstick cooking spray. Broil for 4 minutes on each side or until done. While the lamb cooks, heat a medium saucepan over medium-high heat. Add the remaining oil mixture and cook for 20 seconds, stirring constantly. Stir in broth and bring to a boil. Stir in couscous. Remove from heat, cover and let stand for 5 minutes. Fluff with a fork. Stir in tomatoes, olives and cheese. Serve the couscous mixture with the lamb. Serve with a tossed green salad and fat free dressing. Serves 4.

Nutritional Information: 520 calories; 19.8g fat; 36.2g protein; 36.8g carbohydrate; 3g dietary fiber; 97mg cholesterol; 793mg sodium.

SNACKS AND DESSERTS
(Note: You will need to add these items to the grocery list)

Hot Artichoke-Cheese Dip

2 garlic cloves
1 green onion, cut into pieces
⅓ cup reduced-fat mayonnaise

⅓ cup (1½ oz.) grated Parmigiano-Reggiano cheese, divided
¼ cup (2 oz.) less-fat cream cheese

1 tbsp. fresh lemon juice

¼ tsp. red pepper, crushed

24 (½-oz.) slices baguette, toasted

12 oz. frozen artichoke hearts, thawed and drained

nonstick cooking spray

Preheat oven to 400° F. Place garlic and onion in a food processor and process until finely chopped. Add ¼ cup Parmigiano-Reggiano cheese, mayonnaise, cream cheese, lemon juice and red pepper and process until almost smooth. Pulse artichoke hearts in a blender until coarsely chopped. Spoon the mixture into a 3-cup gratin dish coated with nonstick cooking spray and sprinkle evenly with remaining Parmigiano-Reggiano cheese. Bake at 400° F for 15 minutes or until thoroughly heated and bubbly. Serve hot with baguette. Serves 12.

Nutritional Information: 126 calories; 3.4g fat; 5.1g protein; 20.8g carbohydrate; 2.3g dietary fiber; 7mg cholesterol; 334mg sodium.

Maple Kettle Corn

2 tbsp. canola oil

½ cup unpopped popcorn kernels

¼ cup maple sugar

½ tsp. kosher salt

Heat oil in a 3-quart saucepan over medium-high heat. Add popcorn, sugar and salt to the pan. Cover and cook for 3 minutes or until the kernels begin to pop, shaking the pan frequently. Continue cooking for 2 minutes, shaking pan constantly to prevent burning. When the popping slows down, remove the pan from the heat. Let stand, covered, until all the popping stops. Let cool and store in airtight container. Serves 8.

Nutritional Information: 89 calories; 4g fat; 1.3g protein; 12.3g carbohydrate; 1.8g dietary fiber; 0.0mg cholesterol; 118mg sodium.

Carrot, Apple Ginger Smoothie

½ cup 100% carrot juice, chilled

½ cup unsweetened applesauce

½ cup vanilla fat-free yogurt

1 tsp. fresh lemon juice

½ tsp. fresh ginger, grated and peeled

1 frozen banana, sliced

5 ice cubes (about 2 oz.)

Place all ingredients in a blender and process for 2 minutes or until smooth. Serves 2.

Nutritional Information: 138 calories; 0.1g fat; 4.3g protein; 32.7g carbohydrate; 2.3g dietary fiber; 2mg cholesterol; 79mg sodium.

Cocoa Nib Meringues

½ tsp. cream of tartar
3 large egg whites
½ cup superfine sugar
2 tbsp. unsweetened cocoa
2 tsp. cocoa nibs

1 tsp. instant espresso granules
   or 2 tsp. instant coffee granules
dash of salt
1 tsp. unsweetened cocoa
   (optional)

Preheat oven to 225° F. Line a baking sheet with parchment paper. Place cream of tartar and egg whites in a large bowl and beat with a mixer at high speed until foamy. Gradually add the superfine sugar, 1 tablespoon at a time, beating until stiff peaks form. Add 2 tablespoons unsweetened cocoa, cocoa nibs, instant espresso granules and salt and beat just until blended. Drop the batter by tablespoonfuls onto a prepared baking sheet and bake at 225° for 1 hour. Turn the oven off (do not remove the pan from the oven) and cool the meringues in the closed oven for at least 8 hours or until crisp. Carefully remove the meringues from paper. Sprinkle with 1 teaspoon unsweetened cocoa, if desired, and store in an airtight container. Serves 36.

Nutritional Information: 14 calories; 0.1g fat; 0.4g protein; 3.1g carbohydrate; 0.1g dietary fiber; 0.0mg cholesterol; 9mg sodium.

Spicy Black Bean Hummus

1 garlic clove, peeled
2 tbsp. fresh lemon juice
1 tbsp. tahini (roasted sesame seed
   paste)
1 tsp. ground cumin
¼ tsp. salt
1 (15-oz.) can black beans, rinsed
   and drained

1 small jalapeño pepper, chopped
   (about 2 tbsp.)
dash of red pepper, crushed
2 tsp. extra-virgin olive oil
dash of red pepper, ground
1 (6-oz.) bag pita chips (such as
   Stacy's Simply Naked®)

Place garlic in a food processor and process until finely chopped. Add lemon juice, tahini, cumin, salt, black beans, jalapeño pepper and crushed red pepper and process until smooth. Spoon the bean mixture into a medium bowl and drizzle with extra-virgin olive oil. Sprinkle with ground red pepper and serve with pita chips. Serves 8.

Nutritional Information: 148 calories; 6.2g fat; 4.5g protein; 20.6g carbohydrate; 3.5g dietary fiber; 0.0mg cholesterol; 381mg sodium.

Member Survey

Please answer the following questions to help your leader plan your First Place 4 Health meetings so that your needs might be met in this session. Give this form to your leader at the first group meeting.

Name _____ Birth date _____

Please list those who live in your household.

Name	Relationship	Age

What church do you attend? _____

Are you interested in receiving more information about our church?

       Yes   No

Occupation _____

What talent or area of expertise would you be willing to share with our class?

_____

Why did you join First Place 4 Health?

_____

With notice, would you be willing to lead a Bible study discussion one week?

       Yes   No

Are you comfortable praying out loud? _____

If the assistant leader were absent, would you be willing to assist in weighing in members and possibly evaluating the Live It Trackers?

       Yes   No

Any other comments:

_____

_____

Personal Weight and Measurement Record

Week	Weight	+ or -	Goal this Session	Pounds to goal
1				
2				
3				
4				
5				
6				
7				
8				
9				
10				
11				
12				

Beginning Measurements

Waist _38_   Hips _45_   Thighs _26_   Chest _41¾_

Ending Measurements

Waist _____   Hips _____   Thighs _____   Chest _____

First Place 4 Health
Prayer Partner

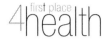

BETTER
TOGETHER
Week
2

SCRIPTURE VERSE TO MEMORIZE FOR WEEK THREE:

Each one should use whatever gift he has received to serve others,
faithfully administering God's grace in its various forms.

1 PETER 4:10

Date: _____

Name: _____

Home Phone: (_____)_____

Work Phone: (_____)_____

Email: _____

Personal Prayer Concerns:

_____
_____
_____
_____
_____
_____
_____

This form is for prayer requests that are personal to you and your journey in First Place 4 Health. Please complete this form and have it ready to turn in when you arrive at your group meeting.

First Place 4 Health
Prayer Partner

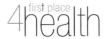

SCRIPTURE VERSE TO MEMORIZE FOR WEEK FOUR:

Be completely humble and gentle; be patient, bearing with one another in love.

EPHESIANS 4:2

Date: _____

Name: _____

Home Phone: (_____) _____

Work Phone: (_____) _____

Email: _____

Personal Prayer Concerns:

_____

_____

_____

_____

_____

_____

_____

This form is for prayer requests that are personal to you and your journey in First Place 4 Health. Please complete this form and have it ready to turn in when you arrive at your group meeting.

First Place 4 Health
Prayer Partner

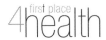

SCRIPTURE VERSE TO MEMORIZE FOR WEEK FIVE:

Let the word of Christ dwell in you richly as you teach and admonish one another with all wisdom, and as you sing psalms, hymns and spiritual songs with gratitude in your hearts to God.

COLOSSIANS 3:16

Date: _____

Name: _____

Home Phone: (_____) _____

Work Phone: (_____) _____

Email: _____

Personal Prayer Concerns:

_____

_____

_____

_____

_____

_____

_____

This form is for prayer requests that are personal to you and your journey in First Place 4 Health. Please complete this form and have it ready to turn in when you arrive at your group meeting.

First Place 4 Health
Prayer Partner

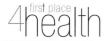

Scripture Verse to Memorize for Week Six:

*This is what the Lord Almighty says: "Administer true justice;
show mercy and compassion to one another."*

Zechariah 7:9

Date: _____

Name: _____

Home Phone: (____) _____

Work Phone: (____) _____

Email: _____

Personal Prayer Concerns:

_____

_____

_____

_____

_____

_____

_____

This form is for prayer requests that are personal to you and your journey in First Place 4 Health. Please complete this form and have it ready to turn in when you arrive at your group meeting.

First Place 4 Health
Prayer Partner

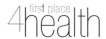

BETTER
TOGETHER
Week
6

Date: _____

Name: _____

Home Phone: (_____)_____

Work Phone: (_____)_____

Email: _____

Personal Prayer Concerns:

_____

_____

_____

_____

_____

_____

_____

This form is for prayer requests that are personal to you and your journey in First Place 4 Health. Please complete this form and have it ready to turn in when you arrive at your group meeting.

First Place 4 Health
Prayer Partner

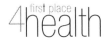

SCRIPTURE VERSE TO MEMORIZE FOR WEEK EIGHT:

*Finally, all of you, live in harmony with one another; be sympathetic,
love as brothers, be compassionate and humble.*

1 PETER 3:8

Date: _____

Name: _____

Home Phone: (_____) _____

Work Phone: (_____) _____

Email: _____

Personal Prayer Concerns:

_____

_____

_____

_____

_____

_____

_____

This form is for prayer requests that are personal to you and your journey in First Place 4 Health. Please complete this form and have it ready to turn in when you arrive at your group meeting.

First Place 4 Health
Prayer Partner

4 first place
health

BETTER
TOGETHER
Week
8

Date: _____

Name: _____

Home Phone: (_____) _____

Work Phone: (_____) _____

Email: _____

Personal Prayer Concerns:

_____

_____

_____

_____

_____

_____

_____

This form is for prayer requests that are personal to you and your journey in First Place 4 Health. Please complete this form and have it ready to turn in when you arrive at your group meeting.

First Place 4 Health
Prayer Partner

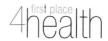

SCRIPTURE VERSE TO MEMORIZE FOR WEEK TEN:

Be devoted to one another in brotherly love. Honor one another above yourselves.

ROMANS 12:10

Date: _____

Name: _____

Home Phone: (_____) _____

Work Phone: (_____) _____

Email: _____

Personal Prayer Concerns:

_____

_____

_____

_____

_____

_____

_____

This form is for prayer requests that are personal to you and your journey in First Place 4 Health. Please complete this form and have it ready to turn in when you arrive at your group meeting.

First Place 4 Health
Prayer Partner

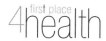

SCRIPTURE VERSE TO MEMORIZE FOR WEEK ELEVEN:

*No one has ever seen God; but if we love one another,
God lives in us and his love is made complete in us*

1 JOHN 4:12

Date: _____

Name: _____

Home Phone: (_____)_____

Work Phone: (_____)_____

Email: _____

Personal Prayer Concerns:

_____

_____

_____

_____

_____

_____

_____

This form is for prayer requests that are personal to you and your journey in First Place 4 Health. Please complete this form and have it ready to turn in when you arrive at your group meeting.

First Place 4 Health
Prayer Partner

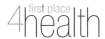

BETTER
TOGETHER
Week
11

Date: _____

Name: _____

Home Phone: (_____) _____

Work Phone: (_____) _____

Email: _____

Personal Prayer Concerns:

_____
_____
_____
_____
_____
_____
_____
_____

This form is for prayer requests that are personal to you and your journey in First Place 4 Health. Please complete this form and have it ready to turn in when you arrive at your group meeting.

Live It Tracker

Name: __Kathleen Hicks__   Loss/gain: _____ lbs.

Date: 9/10/11 Week #: _1_ Calorie Range: _1300_ My food goal for next week: _____

Activity Level: None, < 30 min/day, 30-60 min/day, 60+ min/day My activity goal for next week: _30 min/day_

Group	Daily Calories							
	1300-1400	1500-1600	1700-1800	1900-2000	2100-2200	2300-2400	2500-2600	2700-2800
Fruits	1.5-2 c.	1.5-2 c.	1.5-2 c.	2-2.5 c.	2-2.5 c.	2.5-3.5 c.	3.5-4.5 c.	3.5-4.5 c.
Vegetables	1.5-2 c.	2-2.5 c.	2.5-3 c.	2.5-3 c.	3-3.5 c.	3.5-4.5 c.	4.5-5 c.	4.5-5 c.
Grains	5 oz-eq.	5-6 oz-eq.	6-7 oz-eq.	6-7 oz-eq.	7-8 oz-eq.	8-9 oz-eq.	9-10 oz-eq.	10-11 oz-eq.
Meat & Beans	4 oz-eq.	5 oz-eq.	5-5.5 oz-eq.	5.5-6.5 oz-eq.	6.5-7 oz-eq.	7-7.5 oz-eq.	7-7.5 oz-eq.	7.5-8 oz-eq.
Milk	2-3 c.	3 c.	3 c.	3 c.	3 c.	3 c.	3 c.	3 c.
Healthy Oils	4 tsp.	5 tsp.	5 tsp.	6 tsp.	6 tsp.	7 tsp.	8 tsp.	8 tsp.

Breakfast: 2 eggs- slice Che - c milk Lunch: _1 biscuit-crakz_
Potatoes - Butter - Ezek Bread - Presenza
Dinner: _____   Snack: _____
_____

Day/Date: __

Group	Fruits	Vegetables	Grains	Meat & Beans	Milk	Oils
Goal Amount						
Estimate Your Total						
Increase ⬆ or Decrease? ⬇						

Physical Activity: _____   Spiritual Activity: _____

Steps/Miles/Minutes: _____   _____

Breakfast: _____   Lunch: _____

Dinner: _____   Snack: _____
_____   _____

Day/Date: __

Group	Fruits	Vegetables	Grains	Meat & Beans	Milk	Oils
Goal Amount						
Estimate Your Total						
Increase ⬆ or Decrease? ⬇						

Physical Activity: _____   Spiritual Activity: _____

Steps/Miles/Minutes: _____   _____

Breakfast: _____   Lunch: _____

Dinner: _____   Snack: _____
_____   _____

Day/Date: __

Group	Fruits	Vegetables	Grains	Meat & Beans	Milk	Oils
Goal Amount						
Estimate Your Total						
Increase ⬆ or Decrease? ⬇						

Physical Activity: _____   Spiritual Activity: _____

Steps/Miles/Minutes: _____

Day/Date:

Breakfast: _____   Lunch: _____

Dinner: _____   Snack: _____

Group	Fruits	Vegetables	Grains	Meat & Beans	Milk	Oils
Goal Amount						
Estimate Your Total						
Increase ⇧ or Decrease? ⇩						

Physical Activity: _____   Spiritual Activity: _____

Steps/Miles/Minutes: _____   _____

Day/Date:

Breakfast: _____   Lunch: _____

Dinner: _____   Snack: _____

Group	Fruits	Vegetables	Grains	Meat & Beans	Milk	Oils
Goal Amount						
Estimate Your Total						
Increase ⇧ or Decrease? ⇩						

Physical Activity: _____   Spiritual Activity: _____

Steps/Miles/Minutes: _____   _____

Day/Date:

Breakfast: _____   Lunch: _____

Dinner: _____   Snack: _____

Group	Fruits	Vegetables	Grains	Meat & Beans	Milk	Oils
Goal Amount						
Estimate Your Total						
Increase ⇧ or Decrease? ⇩						

Physical Activity: _____   Spiritual Activity: _____

Steps/Miles/Minutes: _____   _____

Day/Date:

Breakfast: _____   Lunch: _____

Dinner: _____   Snack: _____

Group	Fruits	Vegetables	Grains	Meat & Beans	Milk	Oils
Goal Amount						
Estimate Your Total						
Increase ⇧ or Decrease? ⇩						

Physical Activity: _____   Spiritual Activity: _____

Steps/Miles/Minutes: _____   _____

Live It Tracker

Name: _____ Loss/gain: _____ lbs.

Date: _____ Week #: ____ Calorie Range: _____ My food goal for next week: _____

Activity Level: None, < 30 min/day, 30-60 min/day, 60+ min/day My activity goal for next week: _____

Group	Daily Calories							
	1300-1400	1500-1600	1700-1800	1900-2000	2100-2200	2300-2400	2500-2600	2700-2800
Fruits	1.5-2 c.	1.5-2 c.	1.5-2 c.	2-2.5 c.	2-2.5 c.	2.5-3.5 c.	3.5-4.5 c.	3.5-4.5 c.
Vegetables	1.5-2 c.	2-2.5 c.	2.5-3 c.	2.5-3 c.	3-3.5 c.	3.5-4.5 c.	4.5-5 c.	4.5-5 c.
Grains	5 oz-eq.	5-6 oz-eq.	6-7 oz-eq.	6-7 oz-eq.	7-8 oz-eq.	8-9 oz-eq.	9-10 oz-eq.	10-11 oz-eq.
Meat & Beans	4 oz-eq.	5 oz-eq.	5-5.5 oz-eq.	5.5-6.5 oz-eq.	6.5-7 oz-eq.	7-7.5 oz-eq.	7-7.5 oz-eq.	7.5-8 oz-eq.
Milk	2-3 c.	3 c.	3 c.	3 c.	3 c.	3 c.	3 c.	3 c.
Healthy Oils	4 tsp.	5 tsp.	5 tsp.	6 tsp.	6 tsp.	7 tsp.	8 tsp.	8 tsp.

Day/Date:

Breakfast: _____ Lunch: _____

Dinner: _____ Snack: _____

Group	Fruits	Vegetables	Grains	Meat & Beans	Milk	Oils
Goal Amount						
Estimate Your Total						
Increase ⬆ or Decrease? ⬇						

Physical Activity: _____ Spiritual Activity: _____

Steps/Miles/Minutes: _____ _____

Day/Date:

Breakfast: _____ Lunch: _____

Dinner: _____ Snack: _____

Group	Fruits	Vegetables	Grains	Meat & Beans	Milk	Oils
Goal Amount						
Estimate Your Total						
Increase ⬆ or Decrease? ⬇						

Physical Activity: _____ Spiritual Activity: _____

Steps/Miles/Minutes: _____ _____

Day/Date:

Breakfast: _____ Lunch: _____

Dinner: _____ Snack: _____

Group	Fruits	Vegetables	Grains	Meat & Beans	Milk	Oils
Goal Amount						
Estimate Your Total						
Increase ⬆ or Decrease? ⬇						

Physical Activity: _____ Spiritual Activity: _____

Steps/Miles/Minutes: _____ _____

Day/Date: _____

Breakfast: _____   Lunch: _____

Dinner: _____   Snack: _____

Group	Fruits	Vegetables	Grains	Meat & Beans	Milk	Oils
Goal Amount						
Estimate Your Total						
Increase ⇧ or Decrease? ⇩						

Physical Activity: _____   Spiritual Activity: _____

Steps/Miles/Minutes: _____   _____

Day/Date: _____

Breakfast: _____   Lunch: _____

Dinner: _____   Snack: _____

Group	Fruits	Vegetables	Grains	Meat & Beans	Milk	Oils
Goal Amount						
Estimate Your Total						
Increase ⇧ or Decrease? ⇩						

Physical Activity: _____   Spiritual Activity: _____

Steps/Miles/Minutes: _____   _____

Day/Date: _____

Breakfast: _____   Lunch: _____

Dinner: _____   Snack: _____

Group	Fruits	Vegetables	Grains	Meat & Beans	Milk	Oils
Goal Amount						
Estimate Your Total						
Increase ⇧ or Decrease? ⇩						

Physical Activity: _____   Spiritual Activity: _____

Steps/Miles/Minutes: _____   _____

Day/Date: _____

Breakfast: _____   Lunch: _____

Dinner: _____   Snack: _____

Group	Fruits	Vegetables	Grains	Meat & Beans	Milk	Oils
Goal Amount						
Estimate Your Total						
Increase ⇧ or Decrease? ⇩						

Physical Activity: _____   Spiritual Activity: _____

Steps/Miles/Minutes: _____   _____

Live It Tracker

Name: _____ Loss/gain: _____ lbs.

Date: _____ Week #: _____ Calorie Range: _____ My food goal for next week: _____

Activity Level: None, < 30 min/day, 30-60 min/day, 60+ min/day   My activity goal for next week: _____

Group	Daily Calories							
	1300-1400	1500-1600	1700-1800	1900-2000	2100-2200	2300-2400	2500-2600	2700-2800
Fruits	1.5-2 c.	1.5-2 c.	1.5-2 c.	2-2.5 c.	2-2.5 c.	2.5-3.5 c.	3.5-4.5 c.	3.5-4.5 c.
Vegetables	1.5-2 c.	2-2.5 c.	2.5-3 c.	2.5-3 c.	3-3.5 c.	3.5-4.5 c.	4.5-5 c.	4.5-5 c.
Grains	5 oz-eq.	5-6 oz-eq.	6-7 oz-eq.	6-7 oz-eq.	7-8 oz-eq.	8-9 oz-eq.	9-10 oz-eq.	10-11 oz-eq.
Meat & Beans	4 oz-eq.	5 oz-eq.	5-5.5 oz-eq.	5.5-6.5 oz-eq.	6.5-7 oz-eq.	7-7.5 oz-eq.	7-7.5 oz-eq.	7.5-8 oz-eq.
Milk	2-3 c.	3 c.	3 c.	3 c.	3 c.	3 c.	3 c.	3 c.
Healthy Oils	4 tsp.	5 tsp.	5 tsp.	6 tsp.	6 tsp.	7 tsp.	8 tsp.	8 tsp.

Day/Date:

Breakfast: _____   Lunch: _____

Dinner: _____   Snack: _____

Group	Fruits	Vegetables	Grains	Meat & Beans	Milk	Oils
Goal Amount						
Estimate Your Total						
Increase ⇧ or Decrease? ⇩						

Physical Activity: _____   Spiritual Activity: _____

Steps/Miles/Minutes: _____   _____

Day/Date:

Breakfast: _____   Lunch: _____

Dinner: _____   Snack: _____

Group	Fruits	Vegetables	Grains	Meat & Beans	Milk	Oils
Goal Amount						
Estimate Your Total						
Increase ⇧ or Decrease? ⇩						

Physical Activity: _____   Spiritual Activity: _____

Steps/Miles/Minutes: _____   _____

Day/Date:

Breakfast: _____   Lunch: _____

Dinner: _____   Snack: _____

Group	Fruits	Vegetables	Grains	Meat & Beans	Milk	Oils
Goal Amount						
Estimate Your Total						
Increase ⇧ or Decrease? ⇩						

Physical Activity: _____   Spiritual Activity: _____

Steps/Miles/Minutes: _____   _____

Day/Date:

Breakfast: _____

Lunch: _____

Dinner: _____

Snack: _____

Group	Fruits	Vegetables	Grains	Meat & Beans	Milk	Oils
Goal Amount						
Estimate Your Total						
Increase ⇧ or Decrease? ⇩						

Physical Activity: _____

Spiritual Activity: _____

Steps/Miles/Minutes: _____

_____

Day/Date:

Breakfast: _____

Lunch: _____

Dinner: _____

Snack: _____

Group	Fruits	Vegetables	Grains	Meat & Beans	Milk	Oils
Goal Amount						
Estimate Your Total						
Increase ⇧ or Decrease? ⇩						

Physical Activity: _____

Spiritual Activity: _____

Steps/Miles/Minutes: _____

_____

Day/Date:

Breakfast: _____

Lunch: _____

Dinner: _____

Snack: _____

Group	Fruits	Vegetables	Grains	Meat & Beans	Milk	Oils
Goal Amount						
Estimate Your Total						
Increase ⇧ or Decrease? ⇩						

Physical Activity: _____

Spiritual Activity: _____

Steps/Miles/Minutes: _____

_____

Day/Date:

Breakfast: _____

Lunch: _____

Dinner: _____

Snack: _____

Group	Fruits	Vegetables	Grains	Meat & Beans	Milk	Oils
Goal Amount						
Estimate Your Total						
Increase ⇧ or Decrease? ⇩						

Physical Activity: _____

Spiritual Activity: _____

Steps/Miles/Minutes: _____

Live It Tracker

Name: _____ Loss/gain: _____ lbs.

Date: _____ Week #: _____ Calorie Range: _____ My food goal for next week: _____

Activity Level: None, < 30 min/day, 30-60 min/day, 60+ min/day My activity goal for next week: _____

Group	Daily Calories							
	1300-1400	1500-1600	1700-1800	1900-2000	2100-2200	2300-2400	2500-2600	2700-2800
Fruits	1.5-2 c.	1.5-2 c.	1.5-2 c.	2-2.5 c.	2-2.5 c.	2.5-3.5 c.	3.5-4.5 c.	3.5-4.5 c.
Vegetables	1.5-2 c.	2-2.5 c.	2.5-3 c.	2.5-3 c.	3-3.5 c.	3.5-4.5 c.	4.5-5 c.	4.5-5 c.
Grains	5 oz-eq.	5-6 oz-eq.	6-7 oz-eq.	6-7 oz-eq.	7-8 oz-eq.	8-9 oz-eq.	9-10 oz-eq.	10-11 oz-eq.
Meat & Beans	4 oz-eq.	5 oz-eq.	5-5.5 oz-eq.	5.5-6.5 oz-eq.	6.5-7 oz-eq.	7-7.5 oz-eq.	7-7.5 oz-eq.	7.5-8 oz-eq.
Milk	2-3 c.	3 c.	3 c.	3 c.	3 c.	3 c.	3 c.	3 c.
Healthy Oils	4 tsp.	5 tsp.	5 tsp.	6 tsp.	6 tsp.	7 tsp.	8 tsp.	8 tsp.

Day/Date:

Breakfast: _____ Lunch: _____

Dinner: _____ Snack: _____

Group	Fruits	Vegetables	Grains	Meat & Beans	Milk	Oils
Goal Amount						
Estimate Your Total						
Increase ⇧ or Decrease? ⇩						

Physical Activity: _____ Spiritual Activity: _____

Steps/Miles/Minutes: _____

Day/Date:

Breakfast: _____ Lunch: _____

Dinner: _____ Snack: _____

Group	Fruits	Vegetables	Grains	Meat & Beans	Milk	Oils
Goal Amount						
Estimate Your Total						
Increase ⇧ or Decrease? ⇩						

Physical Activity: _____ Spiritual Activity: _____

Steps/Miles/Minutes: _____

Day/Date:

Breakfast: _____ Lunch: _____

Dinner: _____ Snack: _____

Group	Fruits	Vegetables	Grains	Meat & Beans	Milk	Oils
Goal Amount						
Estimate Your Total						
Increase ⇧ or Decrease? ⇩						

Physical Activity: _____ Spiritual Activity: _____

Steps/Miles/Minutes: _____

Day/Date:

Breakfast: _____ Lunch: _____

Dinner: _____ Snack: _____

Group	Fruits	Vegetables	Grains	Meat & Beans	Milk	Oils
Goal Amount						
Estimate Your Total						
Increase ⇧ or Decrease? ⇩						

Physical Activity: _____ Spiritual Activity: _____

Steps/Miles/Minutes: _____ _____

Day/Date:

Breakfast: _____ Lunch: _____

Dinner: _____ Snack: _____

Group	Fruits	Vegetables	Grains	Meat & Beans	Milk	Oils
Goal Amount						
Estimate Your Total						
Increase ⇧ or Decrease? ⇩						

Physical Activity: _____ Spiritual Activity: _____

Steps/Miles/Minutes: _____ _____

Day/Date:

Breakfast: _____ Lunch: _____

Dinner: _____ Snack: _____

Group	Fruits	Vegetables	Grains	Meat & Beans	Milk	Oils
Goal Amount						
Estimate Your Total						
Increase ⇧ or Decrease? ⇩						

Physical Activity: _____ Spiritual Activity: _____

Steps/Miles/Minutes: _____ _____

Day/Date:

Breakfast: _____ Lunch: _____

Dinner: _____ Snack: _____

Group	Fruits	Vegetables	Grains	Meat & Beans	Milk	Oils
Goal Amount						
Estimate Your Total						
Increase ⇧ or Decrease? ⇩						

Physical Activity: _____ Spiritual Activity: _____

Steps/Miles/Minutes: _____ _____

Live It Tracker

Name: _____ Loss/gain: _____ lbs.

Date: _____ Week #: _____ Calorie Range: _____ My food goal for next week: _____

Activity Level: None, < 30 min/day, 30-60 min/day, 60+ min/day My activity goal for next week: _____

Group	Daily Calories							
	1300-1400	1500-1600	1700-1800	1900-2000	2100-2200	2300-2400	2500-2600	2700-2800
Fruits	1.5-2 c.	1.5-2 c.	1.5-2 c.	2-2.5 c.	2-2.5 c.	2.5-3.5 c.	3.5-4.5 c.	3.5-4.5 c.
Vegetables	1.5-2 c.	2-2.5 c.	2.5-3 c.	2.5-3 c.	3-3.5 c.	3.5-4.5 c.	4.5-5 c.	4.5-5 c.
Grains	5 oz-eq.	5-6 oz-eq.	6-7 oz-eq.	6-7 oz-eq.	7-8 oz-eq.	8-9 oz-eq.	9-10 oz-eq.	10-11 oz-eq.
Meat & Beans	4 oz-eq.	5 oz-eq.	5-5.5 oz-eq.	5.5-6.5 oz-eq.	6.5-7 oz-eq.	7-7.5 oz-eq.	7-7.5 oz-eq.	7.5-8 oz-eq.
Milk	2-3 c.	3 c.	3 c.	3 c.	3 c.	3 c.	3 c.	3 c.
Healthy Oils	4 tsp.	5 tsp.	5 tsp.	6 tsp.	6 tsp.	7 tsp.	8 tsp.	8 tsp.

Day/Date:

Breakfast: _____ Lunch: _____

Dinner: _____ Snack: _____

Group	Fruits	Vegetables	Grains	Meat & Beans	Milk	Oils
Goal Amount						
Estimate Your Total						
Increase ⇧ or Decrease? ⇩						

Physical Activity: _____ Spiritual Activity: _____

Steps/Miles/Minutes: _____ _____

Day/Date:

Breakfast: _____ Lunch: _____

Dinner: _____ Snack: _____

Group	Fruits	Vegetables	Grains	Meat & Beans	Milk	Oils
Goal Amount						
Estimate Your Total						
Increase ⇧ or Decrease? ⇩						

Physical Activity: _____ Spiritual Activity: _____

Steps/Miles/Minutes: _____ _____

Day/Date:

Breakfast: _____ Lunch: _____

Dinner: _____ Snack: _____

Group	Fruits	Vegetables	Grains	Meat & Beans	Milk	Oils
Goal Amount						
Estimate Your Total						
Increase ⇧ or Decrease? ⇩						

Physical Activity: _____ Spiritual Activity: _____

Steps/Miles/Minutes: _____ _____

Day/Date: _____

Breakfast: _____ Lunch: _____

Dinner: _____ Snack: _____

Group	Fruits	Vegetables	Grains	Meat & Beans	Milk	Oils
Goal Amount						
Estimate Your Total						
Increase ⇧ or Decrease? ⇩						

Physical Activity: _____ Spiritual Activity: _____

Steps/Miles/Minutes: _____ _____

Day/Date: _____

Breakfast: _____ Lunch: _____

Dinner: _____ Snack: _____

Group	Fruits	Vegetables	Grains	Meat & Beans	Milk	Oils
Goal Amount						
Estimate Your Total						
Increase ⇧ or Decrease? ⇩						

Physical Activity: _____ Spiritual Activity: _____

Steps/Miles/Minutes: _____ _____

Day/Date: _____

Breakfast: _____ Lunch: _____

Dinner: _____ Snack: _____

Group	Fruits	Vegetables	Grains	Meat & Beans	Milk	Oils
Goal Amount						
Estimate Your Total						
Increase ⇧ or Decrease? ⇩						

Physical Activity: _____ Spiritual Activity: _____

Steps/Miles/Minutes: _____ _____

Day/Date: _____

Breakfast: _____ Lunch: _____

Dinner: _____ Snack: _____

Group	Fruits	Vegetables	Grains	Meat & Beans	Milk	Oils
Goal Amount						
Estimate Your Total						
Increase ⇧ or Decrease? ⇩						

Physical Activity: _____ Spiritual Activity: _____

Steps/Miles/Minutes: _____ _____

Live It Tracker

Name: _____ Loss/gain: _____ lbs.

Date: _____ Week #: ____ Calorie Range: _____ My food goal for next week: _____

Activity Level: None, < 30 min/day, 30-60 min/day, 60+ min/day My activity goal for next week: _____

Group	Daily Calories							
	1300-1400	1500-1600	1700-1800	1900-2000	2100-2200	2300-2400	2500-2600	2700-2800
Fruits	1.5-2 c.	1.5-2 c.	1.5-2 c.	2-2.5 c.	2-2.5 c.	2.5-3.5 c.	3.5-4.5 c.	3.5-4.5 c.
Vegetables	1.5-2 c.	2-2.5 c.	2.5-3 c.	2.5-3 c.	3-3.5 c.	3.5-4.5 c.	4.5-5 c.	4.5-5 c.
Grains	5 oz-eq.	5-6 oz-eq.	6-7 oz-eq.	6-7 oz-eq.	7-8 oz-eq.	8-9 oz-eq.	9-10 oz-eq.	10-11 oz-eq.
Meat & Beans	4 oz-eq.	5 oz-eq.	5-5.5 oz-eq.	5.5-6.5 oz-eq.	6.5-7 oz-eq.	7-7.5 oz-eq.	7-7.5 oz-eq.	7.5-8 oz-eq.
Milk	2-3 c.	3 c.	3 c.	3 c.	3 c.	3 c.	3 c.	3 c.
Healthy Oils	4 tsp.	5 tsp.	5 tsp.	6 tsp.	6 tsp.	7 tsp.	8 tsp.	8 tsp.

Day/Date: _____

Breakfast: _____ Lunch: _____

Dinner: _____ Snack: _____

Group	Fruits	Vegetables	Grains	Meat & Beans	Milk	Oils
Goal Amount						
Estimate Your Total						
Increase ⇧ or Decrease? ⇩						

Physical Activity: _____ Spiritual Activity: _____

Steps/Miles/Minutes: _____ _____

Day/Date: _____

Breakfast: _____ Lunch: _____

Dinner: _____ Snack: _____

Group	Fruits	Vegetables	Grains	Meat & Beans	Milk	Oils
Goal Amount						
Estimate Your Total						
Increase ⇧ or Decrease? ⇩						

Physical Activity: _____ Spiritual Activity: _____

Steps/Miles/Minutes: _____ _____

Day/Date: _____

Breakfast: _____ Lunch: _____

Dinner: _____ Snack: _____

Group	Fruits	Vegetables	Grains	Meat & Beans	Milk	Oils
Goal Amount						
Estimate Your Total						
Increase ⇧ or Decrease? ⇩						

Physical Activity: _____ Spiritual Activity: _____

Steps/Miles/Minutes: _____ _____

Day/Date:

Breakfast: _____ Lunch: _____

Dinner: _____ Snack: _____

Group	Fruits	Vegetables	Grains	Meat & Beans	Milk	Oils
Goal Amount						
Estimate Your Total						
Increase ⬆ or Decrease? ⬇						

Physical Activity: _____ Spiritual Activity: _____

Steps/Miles/Minutes: _____

Day/Date:

Breakfast: _____ Lunch: _____

Dinner: _____ Snack: _____

Group	Fruits	Vegetables	Grains	Meat & Beans	Milk	Oils
Goal Amount						
Estimate Your Total						
Increase ⬆ or Decrease? ⬇						

Physical Activity: _____ Spiritual Activity: _____

Steps/Miles/Minutes: _____

Day/Date:

Breakfast: _____ Lunch: _____

Dinner: _____ Snack: _____

Group	Fruits	Vegetables	Grains	Meat & Beans	Milk	Oils
Goal Amount						
Estimate Your Total						
Increase ⬆ or Decrease? ⬇						

Physical Activity: _____ Spiritual Activity: _____

Steps/Miles/Minutes: _____

Day/Date:

Breakfast: _____ Lunch: _____

Dinner: _____ Snack: _____

Group	Fruits	Vegetables	Grains	Meat & Beans	Milk	Oils
Goal Amount						
Estimate Your Total						
Increase ⬆ or Decrease? ⬇						

Physical Activity: _____ Spiritual Activity: _____

Steps/Miles/Minutes: _____

Live It Tracker

Name: _____ Loss/gain: _____ lbs.

Date: _____ Week #: _____ Calorie Range: _____ My food goal for next week: _____

Activity Level: None, < 30 min/day, 30-60 min/day, 60+ min/day My activity goal for next week: _____

Group	Daily Calories							
	1300-1400	1500-1600	1700-1800	1900-2000	2100-2200	2300-2400	2500-2600	2700-2800
Fruits	1.5-2 c.	1.5-2 c.	1.5-2 c.	2-2.5 c.	2-2.5 c.	2.5-3.5 c.	3.5-4.5 c.	3.5-4.5 c.
Vegetables	1.5-2 c.	2-2.5 c.	2.5-3 c.	2.5-3 c.	3-3.5 c.	3.5-4.5 c.	4.5-5 c.	4.5-5 c.
Grains	5 oz-eq.	5-6 oz-eq.	6-7 oz-eq.	6-7 oz-eq.	7-8 oz-eq.	8-9 oz-eq.	9-10 oz-eq.	10-11 oz-eq.
Meat & Beans	4 oz-eq.	5 oz-eq.	5-5.5 oz-eq.	5.5-6.5 oz-eq.	6.5-7 oz-eq.	7-7.5 oz-eq.	7-7.5 oz-eq.	7.5-8 oz-eq.
Milk	2-3 c.	3 c.	3 c.	3 c.	3 c.	3 c.	3 c.	3 c.
Healthy Oils	4 tsp.	5 tsp.	5 tsp.	6 tsp.	6 tsp.	7 tsp.	8 tsp.	8 tsp.

Day/Date:

Breakfast: _____ Lunch: _____

Dinner: _____ Snack: _____

Group	Fruits	Vegetables	Grains	Meat & Beans	Milk	Oils
Goal Amount						
Estimate Your Total						
Increase ⇧ or Decrease? ⇩						

Physical Activity: _____ Spiritual Activity: _____

Steps/Miles/Minutes: _____ _____

Day/Date:

Breakfast: _____ Lunch: _____

Dinner: _____ Snack: _____

Group	Fruits	Vegetables	Grains	Meat & Beans	Milk	Oils
Goal Amount						
Estimate Your Total						
Increase ⇧ or Decrease? ⇩						

Physical Activity: _____ Spiritual Activity: _____

Steps/Miles/Minutes: _____ _____

Day/Date:

Breakfast: _____ Lunch: _____

Dinner: _____ Snack: _____

Group	Fruits	Vegetables	Grains	Meat & Beans	Milk	Oils
Goal Amount						
Estimate Your Total						
Increase ⇧ or Decrease? ⇩						

Physical Activity: _____ Spiritual Activity: _____

Steps/Miles/Minutes: _____

Day/Date:

Breakfast: _____

Lunch: _____

Dinner: _____

Snack: _____

Group	Fruits	Vegetables	Grains	Meat & Beans	Milk	Oils
Goal Amount						
Estimate Your Total						
Increase ⇧ or Decrease? ⇩						

Physical Activity: _____

Spiritual Activity: _____

Steps/Miles/Minutes: _____

Day/Date:

Breakfast: _____

Lunch: _____

Dinner: _____

Snack: _____

Group	Fruits	Vegetables	Grains	Meat & Beans	Milk	Oils
Goal Amount						
Estimate Your Total						
Increase ⇧ or Decrease? ⇩						

Physical Activity: _____

Spiritual Activity: _____

Steps/Miles/Minutes: _____

Day/Date:

Breakfast: _____

Lunch: _____

Dinner: _____

Snack: _____

Group	Fruits	Vegetables	Grains	Meat & Beans	Milk	Oils
Goal Amount						
Estimate Your Total						
Increase ⇧ or Decrease? ⇩						

Physical Activity: _____

Spiritual Activity: _____

Steps/Miles/Minutes: _____

Day/Date:

Breakfast: _____

Lunch: _____

Dinner: _____

Snack: _____

Group	Fruits	Vegetables	Grains	Meat & Beans	Milk	Oils
Goal Amount						
Estimate Your Total						
Increase ⇧ or Decrease? ⇩						

Physical Activity: _____

Spiritual Activity: _____

Steps/Miles/Minutes: _____

Live It Tracker

Name: _____ Loss/gain: _____ lbs.

Date: _____ Week #: _____ Calorie Range: _____ My food goal for next week: _____

Activity Level: None, < 30 min/day, 30-60 min/day, 60+ min/day My activity goal for next week: _____

Group	Daily Calories							
	1300-1400	1500-1600	1700-1800	1900-2000	2100-2200	2300-2400	2500-2600	2700-2800
Fruits	1.5-2 c.	1.5-2 c.	1.5-2 c.	2-2.5 c.	2-2.5 c.	2.5-3.5 c.	3.5-4.5 c.	3.5-4.5 c.
Vegetables	1.5-2 c.	2-2.5 c.	2.5-3 c.	2.5-3 c.	3-3.5 c.	3.5-4.5 c.	4.5-5 c.	4.5-5 c.
Grains	5 oz-eq.	5-6 oz-eq.	6-7 oz-eq.	6-7 oz-eq.	7-8 oz-eq.	8-9 oz-eq.	9-10 oz-eq.	10-11 oz-eq.
Meat & Beans	4 oz-eq.	5 oz-eq.	5-5.5 oz-eq.	5.5-6.5 oz-eq.	6.5-7 oz-eq.	7-7.5 oz-eq.	7-7.5 oz-eq.	7.5-8 oz-eq.
Milk	2-3 c.	3 c.	3 c.	3 c.	3 c.	3 c.	3 c.	3 c.
Healthy Oils	4 tsp.	5 tsp.	5 tsp.	6 tsp.	6 tsp.	7 tsp.	8 tsp.	8 tsp.

Day/Date:

Breakfast: _____ Lunch: _____

Dinner: _____ Snack: _____

Group	Fruits	Vegetables	Grains	Meat & Beans	Milk	Oils
Goal Amount						
Estimate Your Total						
Increase ⇧ or Decrease? ⇩						

Physical Activity: _____ Spiritual Activity: _____

Steps/Miles/Minutes: _____ _____

Day/Date:

Breakfast: _____ Lunch: _____

Dinner: _____ Snack: _____

Group	Fruits	Vegetables	Grains	Meat & Beans	Milk	Oils
Goal Amount						
Estimate Your Total						
Increase ⇧ or Decrease? ⇩						

Physical Activity: _____ Spiritual Activity: _____

Steps/Miles/Minutes: _____ _____

Day/Date:

Breakfast: _____ Lunch: _____

Dinner: _____ Snack: _____

Group	Fruits	Vegetables	Grains	Meat & Beans	Milk	Oils
Goal Amount						
Estimate Your Total						
Increase ⇧ or Decrease? ⇩						

Physical Activity: _____ Spiritual Activity: _____

Steps/Miles/Minutes: _____ _____

Day/Date:

Breakfast: _____   Lunch: _____
_____

Dinner: _____   Snack: _____
_____

Group	Fruits	Vegetables	Grains	Meat & Beans	Milk	Oils
Goal Amount						
Estimate Your Total						
Increase ⇧ or Decrease? ⇩						

Physical Activity: _____   Spiritual Activity: _____
Steps/Miles/Minutes: _____   _____

Day/Date:

Breakfast: _____   Lunch: _____
_____   _____

Dinner: _____   Snack: _____
_____   _____

Group	Fruits	Vegetables	Grains	Meat & Beans	Milk	Oils
Goal Amount						
Estimate Your Total						
Increase ⇧ or Decrease? ⇩						

Physical Activity: _____   Spiritual Activity: _____
Steps/Miles/Minutes: _____   _____

Day/Date:

Breakfast: _____   Lunch: _____
_____

Dinner: _____   Snack: _____
_____

Group	Fruits	Vegetables	Grains	Meat & Beans	Milk	Oils
Goal Amount						
Estimate Your Total						
Increase ⇧ or Decrease? ⇩						

Physical Activity: _____   Spiritual Activity: _____
Steps/Miles/Minutes: _____   _____

Day/Date:

Breakfast: _____   Lunch: _____
_____

Dinner: _____   Snack: _____
_____

Group	Fruits	Vegetables	Grains	Meat & Beans	Milk	Oils
Goal Amount						
Estimate Your Total						
Increase ⇧ or Decrease? ⇩						

Physical Activity: _____   Spiritual Activity: _____
Steps/Miles/Minutes: _____   _____

Live It Tracker

Name: _____ Loss/gain: _____ lbs.

Date: _____ Week #: _____ Calorie Range: _____ My food goal for next week: _____

Activity Level: None, < 30 min/day, 30-60 min/day, 60+ min/day My activity goal for next week: _____

Group	Daily Calories							
	1300-1400	1500-1600	1700-1800	1900-2000	2100-2200	2300-2400	2500-2600	2700-2800
Fruits	1.5-2 c.	1.5-2 c.	1.5-2 c.	2-2.5 c.	2-2.5 c.	2.5-3.5 c.	3.5-4.5 c.	3.5-4.5 c.
Vegetables	1.5-2 c.	2-2.5 c.	2.5-3 c.	2.5-3 c.	3-3.5 c.	3.5-4.5 c.	4.5-5 c.	4.5-5 c.
Grains	5 oz-eq.	5-6 oz-eq.	6-7 oz-eq.	6-7 oz-eq.	7-8 oz-eq.	8-9 oz-eq.	9-10 oz-eq.	10-11 oz-eq.
Meat & Beans	4 oz-eq.	5 oz-eq.	5-5.5 oz-eq.	5.5-6.5 oz-eq.	6.5-7 oz-eq.	7-7.5 oz-eq.	7-7.5 oz-eq.	7.5-8 oz-eq.
Milk	2-3 c.	3 c.	3 c.	3 c.	3 c.	3 c.	3 c.	3 c.
Healthy Oils	4 tsp.	5 tsp.	5 tsp.	6 tsp.	6 tsp.	7 tsp.	8 tsp.	8 tsp.

Day/Date: _____

Breakfast: _____   Lunch: _____

Dinner: _____   Snack: _____

Group	Fruits	Vegetables	Grains	Meat & Beans	Milk	Oils
Goal Amount						
Estimate Your Total						
Increase ⇧ or Decrease? ⇩						

Physical Activity: _____   Spiritual Activity: _____

Steps/Miles/Minutes: _____   _____

Day/Date: _____

Breakfast: _____   Lunch: _____

Dinner: _____   Snack: _____

Group	Fruits	Vegetables	Grains	Meat & Beans	Milk	Oils
Goal Amount						
Estimate Your Total						
Increase ⇧ or Decrease? ⇩						

Physical Activity: _____   Spiritual Activity: _____

Steps/Miles/Minutes: _____   _____

Day/Date: _____

Breakfast: _____   Lunch: _____

Dinner: _____   Snack: _____

Group	Fruits	Vegetables	Grains	Meat & Beans	Milk	Oils
Goal Amount						
Estimate Your Total						
Increase ⇧ or Decrease? ⇩						

Physical Activity: _____   Spiritual Activity: _____

Steps/Miles/Minutes: _____   _____

Day/Date: _____

Breakfast: _____ Lunch: _____

Dinner: _____ Snack: _____

Group	Fruits	Vegetables	Grains	Meat & Beans	Milk	Oils
Goal Amount						
Estimate Your Total						
Increase ⇧ or Decrease? ⇩						

Physical Activity: _____ Spiritual Activity: _____

Steps/Miles/Minutes: _____ _____

Day/Date: _____

Breakfast: _____ Lunch: _____

Dinner: _____ Snack: _____

Group	Fruits	Vegetables	Grains	Meat & Beans	Milk	Oils
Goal Amount						
Estimate Your Total						
Increase ⇧ or Decrease? ⇩						

Physical Activity: _____ Spiritual Activity: _____

Steps/Miles/Minutes: _____ _____

Day/Date: _____

Breakfast: _____ Lunch: _____

Dinner: _____ Snack: _____

Group	Fruits	Vegetables	Grains	Meat & Beans	Milk	Oils
Goal Amount						
Estimate Your Total						
Increase ⇧ or Decrease? ⇩						

Physical Activity: _____ Spiritual Activity: _____

Steps/Miles/Minutes: _____ _____

Day/Date: _____

Breakfast: _____ Lunch: _____

Dinner: _____ Snack: _____

Group	Fruits	Vegetables	Grains	Meat & Beans	Milk	Oils
Goal Amount						
Estimate Your Total						
Increase ⇧ or Decrease? ⇩						

Physical Activity: _____ Spiritual Activity: _____

Steps/Miles/Minutes: _____ _____

Live It Tracker

Name: _____ Loss/gain: _____ lbs.

Date: _____ Week #: _____ Calorie Range: _____ My food goal for next week: _____

Activity Level: None, < 30 min/day, 30-60 min/day, 60+ min/day My activity goal for next week: _____

Group	Daily Calories							
	1300-1400	1500-1600	1700-1800	1900-2000	2100-2200	2300-2400	2500-2600	2700-2800
Fruits	1.5-2 c.	1.5-2 c.	1.5-2 c.	2-2.5 c.	2-2.5 c.	2.5-3.5 c.	3.5-4.5 c.	3.5-4.5 c.
Vegetables	1.5-2 c.	2-2.5 c.	2.5-3 c.	2.5-3 c.	3-3.5 c.	3.5-4.5 c.	4.5-5 c.	4.5-5 c.
Grains	5 oz-eq.	5-6 oz-eq.	6-7 oz-eq.	6-7 oz-eq.	7-8 oz-eq.	8-9 oz-eq.	9-10 oz-eq.	10-11 oz-eq.
Meat & Beans	4 oz-eq.	5 oz-eq.	5-5.5 oz-eq.	5.5-6.5 oz-eq.	6.5-7 oz-eq.	7-7.5 oz-eq.	7-7.5 oz-eq.	7.5-8 oz-eq.
Milk	2-3 c.	3 c.	3 c.	3 c.	3 c.	3 c.	3 c.	3 c.
Healthy Oils	4 tsp.	5 tsp.	5 tsp.	6 tsp.	6 tsp.	7 tsp.	8 tsp.	8 tsp.

Day/Date: _____

Breakfast: _____ Lunch: _____

Dinner: _____ Snack: _____

Group	Fruits	Vegetables	Grains	Meat & Beans	Milk	Oils
Goal Amount						
Estimate Your Total						
Increase ⇧ or Decrease? ⇩						

Physical Activity: _____ Spiritual Activity: _____

Steps/Miles/Minutes: _____ _____

Day/Date: _____

Breakfast: _____ Lunch: _____

Dinner: _____ Snack: _____

Group	Fruits	Vegetables	Grains	Meat & Beans	Milk	Oils
Goal Amount						
Estimate Your Total						
Increase ⇧ or Decrease? ⇩						

Physical Activity: _____ Spiritual Activity: _____

Steps/Miles/Minutes: _____ _____

Day/Date: _____

Breakfast: _____ Lunch: _____

Dinner: _____ Snack: _____

Group	Fruits	Vegetables	Grains	Meat & Beans	Milk	Oils
Goal Amount						
Estimate Your Total						
Increase ⇧ or Decrease? ⇩						

Physical Activity: _____ Spiritual Activity: _____

Steps/Miles/Minutes: _____ _____

Day/Date: _____

Breakfast: _____ Lunch: _____

Dinner: _____ Snack: _____

Group	Fruits	Vegetables	Grains	Meat & Beans	Milk	Oils
Goal Amount						
Estimate Your Total						
Increase ⇧ or Decrease? ⇩						

Physical Activity: _____ Spiritual Activity: _____

Steps/Miles/Minutes: _____ _____

Day/Date: _____

Breakfast: _____ Lunch: _____

Dinner: _____ Snack: _____

Group	Fruits	Vegetables	Grains	Meat & Beans	Milk	Oils
Goal Amount						
Estimate Your Total						
Increase ⇧ or Decrease? ⇩						

Physical Activity: _____ Spiritual Activity: _____

Steps/Miles/Minutes: _____ _____

Day/Date: _____

Breakfast: _____ Lunch: _____

Dinner: _____ Snack: _____

Group	Fruits	Vegetables	Grains	Meat & Beans	Milk	Oils
Goal Amount						
Estimate Your Total						
Increase ⇧ or Decrease? ⇩						

Physical Activity: _____ Spiritual Activity: _____

Steps/Miles/Minutes: _____ _____

Day/Date: _____

Breakfast: _____ Lunch: _____

Dinner: _____ Snack: _____

Group	Fruits	Vegetables	Grains	Meat & Beans	Milk	Oils
Goal Amount						
Estimate Your Total						
Increase ⇧ or Decrease? ⇩						

Physical Activity: _____ Spiritual Activity: _____

Steps/Miles/Minutes: _____ _____

Live It Tracker

Name: _____ Loss/gain: _____ lbs.

Date: _____ Week #: ____ Calorie Range: _____ My food goal for next week: _____

Activity Level: None, < 30 min/day, 30-60 min/day, 60+ min/day My activity goal for next week: _____

Group	Daily Calories							
	1300-1400	1500-1600	1700-1800	1900-2000	2100-2200	2300-2400	2500-2600	2700-2800
Fruits	1.5-2 c.	1.5-2 c.	1.5-2 c.	2-2.5 c.	2-2.5 c.	2.5-3.5 c.	3.5-4.5 c.	3.5-4.5 c.
Vegetables	1.5-2 c.	2-2.5 c.	2.5-3 c.	2.5-3 c.	3-3.5 c.	3.5-4.5 c.	4.5-5 c.	4.5-5 c.
Grains	5 oz-eq.	5-6 oz-eq.	6-7 oz-eq.	6-7 oz-eq.	7-8 oz-eq.	8-9 oz-eq.	9-10 oz-eq.	10-11 oz-eq.
Meat & Beans	4 oz-eq.	5 oz-eq.	5-5.5 oz-eq.	5.5-6.5 oz-eq.	6.5-7 oz-eq.	7-7.5 oz-eq.	7-7.5 oz-eq.	7.5-8 oz-eq.
Milk	2-3 c.	3 c.	3 c.	3 c.	3 c.	3 c.	3 c.	3 c.
Healthy Oils	4 tsp.	5 tsp.	5 tsp.	6 tsp.	6 tsp.	7 tsp.	8 tsp.	8 tsp.

Day/Date: _____

Breakfast: _____ Lunch: _____

Dinner: _____ Snack: _____

Group	Fruits	Vegetables	Grains	Meat & Beans	Milk	Oils
Goal Amount						
Estimate Your Total						
Increase ⇧ or Decrease? ⇩						

Physical Activity: _____ Spiritual Activity: _____

Steps/Miles/Minutes: _____

Day/Date: _____

Breakfast: _____ Lunch: _____

Dinner: _____ Snack: _____

Group	Fruits	Vegetables	Grains	Meat & Beans	Milk	Oils
Goal Amount						
Estimate Your Total						
Increase ⇧ or Decrease? ⇩						

Physical Activity: _____ Spiritual Activity: _____

Steps/Miles/Minutes: _____

Day/Date: _____

Breakfast: _____ Lunch: _____

Dinner: _____ Snack: _____

Group	Fruits	Vegetables	Grains	Meat & Beans	Milk	Oils
Goal Amount						
Estimate Your Total						
Increase ⇧ or Decrease? ⇩						

Physical Activity: _____ Spiritual Activity: _____

Steps/Miles/Minutes: _____

Day/Date: _____

Breakfast: _____ Lunch: _____

Dinner: _____ Snack: _____

Group	Fruits	Vegetables	Grains	Meat & Beans	Milk	Oils
Goal Amount						
Estimate Your Total						
Increase ⇧ or Decrease? ⇩						

Physical Activity: _____ Spiritual Activity: _____

Steps/Miles/Minutes: _____ _____

Day/Date: _____

Breakfast: _____ Lunch: _____

Dinner: _____ Snack: _____

Group	Fruits	Vegetables	Grains	Meat & Beans	Milk	Oils
Goal Amount						
Estimate Your Total						
Increase ⇧ or Decrease? ⇩						

Physical Activity: _____ Spiritual Activity: _____

Steps/Miles/Minutes: _____ _____

Day/Date: _____

Breakfast: _____ Lunch: _____

Dinner: _____ Snack: _____

Group	Fruits	Vegetables	Grains	Meat & Beans	Milk	Oils
Goal Amount						
Estimate Your Total						
Increase ⇧ or Decrease? ⇩						

Physical Activity: _____ Spiritual Activity: _____

Steps/Miles/Minutes: _____ _____

Day/Date: _____

Breakfast: _____ Lunch: _____

Dinner: _____ Snack: _____

Group	Fruits	Vegetables	Grains	Meat & Beans	Milk	Oils
Goal Amount						
Estimate Your Total						
Increase ⇧ or Decrease? ⇩						

Physical Activity: _____ Spiritual Activity: _____

Steps/Miles/Minutes: _____ _____

Live It Tracker

Name: _____ Loss/gain: _____ lbs.

Date: _____ Week #: _____ Calorie Range: _____ My food goal for next week: _____

Activity Level: None, < 30 min/day, 30-60 min/day, 60+ min/day My activity goal for next week: _____

Group	Daily Calories							
	1300-1400	1500-1600	1700-1800	1900-2000	2100-2200	2300-2400	2500-2600	2700-2800
Fruits	1.5-2 c.	1.5-2 c.	1.5-2 c.	2-2.5 c.	2-2.5 c.	2.5-3.5 c.	3.5-4.5 c.	3.5-4.5 c.
Vegetables	1.5-2 c.	2-2.5 c.	2.5-3 c.	2.5-3 c.	3-3.5 c.	3.5-4.5 c.	4.5-5 c.	4.5-5 c.
Grains	5 oz-eq.	5-6 oz-eq.	6-7 oz-eq.	6-7 oz-eq.	7-8 oz-eq.	8-9 oz-eq.	9-10 oz-eq.	10-11 oz-eq.
Meat & Beans	4 oz-eq.	5 oz-eq.	5-5.5 oz-eq.	5.5-6.5 oz-eq.	6.5-7 oz-eq.	7-7.5 oz-eq.	7-7.5 oz-eq.	7.5-8 oz-eq.
Milk	2-3 c.	3 c.	3 c.	3 c.	3 c.	3 c.	3 c.	3 c.
Healthy Oils	4 tsp.	5 tsp.	5 tsp.	6 tsp.	6 tsp.	7 tsp.	8 tsp.	8 tsp.

Day/Date:

Breakfast: _____   Lunch: _____

Dinner: _____   Snack: _____

Group	Fruits	Vegetables	Grains	Meat & Beans	Milk	Oils
Goal Amount						
Estimate Your Total						
Increase ⇧ or Decrease? ⇩						

Physical Activity: _____   Spiritual Activity: _____

Steps/Miles/Minutes: _____   _____

Day/Date:

Breakfast: _____   Lunch: _____

Dinner: _____   Snack: _____

Group	Fruits	Vegetables	Grains	Meat & Beans	Milk	Oils
Goal Amount						
Estimate Your Total						
Increase ⇧ or Decrease? ⇩						

Physical Activity: _____   Spiritual Activity: _____

Steps/Miles/Minutes: _____   _____

Day/Date:

Breakfast: _____   Lunch: _____

Dinner: _____   Snack: _____

Group	Fruits	Vegetables	Grains	Meat & Beans	Milk	Oils
Goal Amount						
Estimate Your Total						
Increase ⇧ or Decrease? ⇩						

Physical Activity: _____   Spiritual Activity: _____

Steps/Miles/Minutes: _____   _____

Day/Date: _____

Breakfast: _____ Lunch: _____

Dinner: _____ Snack: _____

Group	Fruits	Vegetables	Grains	Meat & Beans	Milk	Oils
Goal Amount						
Estimate Your Total						
Increase ⇧ or Decrease? ⇩						

Physical Activity: _____ Spiritual Activity: _____

Steps/Miles/Minutes: _____ _____

Day/Date: _____

Breakfast: _____ Lunch: _____

Dinner: _____ Snack: _____

Group	Fruits	Vegetables	Grains	Meat & Beans	Milk	Oils
Goal Amount						
Estimate Your Total						
Increase ⇧ or Decrease? ⇩						

Physical Activity: _____ Spiritual Activity: _____

Steps/Miles/Minutes: _____ _____

Day/Date: _____

Breakfast: _____ Lunch: _____

Dinner: _____ Snack: _____

Group	Fruits	Vegetables	Grains	Meat & Beans	Milk	Oils
Goal Amount						
Estimate Your Total						
Increase ⇧ or Decrease? ⇩						

Physical Activity: _____ Spiritual Activity: _____

Steps/Miles/Minutes: _____ _____

Day/Date: _____

Breakfast: _____ Lunch: _____

Dinner: _____ Snack: _____

Group	Fruits	Vegetables	Grains	Meat & Beans	Milk	Oils
Goal Amount						
Estimate Your Total						
Increase ⇧ or Decrease? ⇩						

Physical Activity: _____ Spiritual Activity: _____

Steps/Miles/Minutes: _____ _____

let's count our miles!

Join the 100-Mile Club this Session

Can't walk that mile yet? Don't be discouraged! There are exercises you can do to strengthen your body and burn those extra calories. Keep a record on your Live It Tracker of the number of minutes you do these common physical activities, convert those minutes to miles following the chart below, and then mark off each mile you have completed on the chart found on the back of the back cover. Report your miles to your 100-Mile Club representative when you first arrive each week. Remember, you are not competing with anyone else . . . just yourself. Your job is to strive to reach 100 miles before the last meeting in this session. You can do it—just keep on moving!

Walking

slowly, 2 mph	30 min. = 156 cal. = 1 mile
moderately, 3 mph	20 min. = 156 cal. = 1 mile
very briskly, 4 mph	15 min. = 156 cal. = 1 mile
speed walking	10 min. = 156 cal. = 1 mile
up stairs	13 min. = 159 cal. = 1 mile

Running/Jogging
10 min. = 156 cal. = 1 mile

Cycling Outdoors

slowly, <10 mph	20 min. = 156 cal. = 1 mile
light effort, 10-12 mph	12 min. = 156 cal. = 1 mile
moderate effort, 12-14 mph	10 min. = 156 cal. = 1 mile
vigorous effort, 14-16 mph	7.5 min. = 156 cal. = 1 mile
very fast, 16-19 mph	6.5 min. = 152 cal. = 1 mile

Sports Activities

Playing tennis (singles)	10 min. = 156 cal. = 1 mile
Swimming	
light to moderate effort	11 min. = 152 cal. = 1 mile
fast, vigorous effort	7.5 min. = 156 cal. = 1 mile
Softball	15 min. = 156 cal. = 1 mile
Golf	20 min. = 156 cal = 1 mile
Rollerblading	6.5 min. = 152 cal. = 1 mile
Ice skating	11 min. = 152 cal. = 1 mile

Jumping rope	7.5 min. = 156 cal. = 1 mile
Basketball	12 min. = 156 cal. = 1 mile
Soccer (casual)	15 min. = 159 cal. = 1 mile

Around the House

Mowing grass	22 min. = 156 cal. = 1 mile
Mopping, sweeping, vacuuming	19.5 min. = 155 cal. = 1 mile
Cooking	40 min. =160 cal. = 1 mile
Gardening	19 min. = 156 cal. = 1 mile
Housework (general)	35 min. = 156 cal. = 1 mile
Ironing	45 min. = 153 cal. = 1 mile
Raking leaves	25 min. = 150 cal. = 1 mile
Washing car	23 min. = 156 cal. = 1 mile
Washing dishes	45 min. = 153 cal. = 1 mile

At the Gym

Stair machine	8.5 min. = 155 cal. = 1 mile
Stationary bike	
slowly, 10 mph	30 min. = 156 cal. = 1 mile
moderately, 10-13 mph	15 min. = 156 cal. = 1 mile
vigorously, 13-16 mph	7.5 min. = 156 cal. = 1 mile
briskly, 16-19 mph	6.5 min. = 156 cal. = 1 mile
Elliptical trainer	12 min. = 156 cal. = 1 mile
Weight machines (used vigorously)	13 min. = 152 cal.=1 mile
Aerobics	
low impact	15 min. = 156 cal. = 1 mile
high impact	12 min. = 156 cal. = 1 mile
water	20 min. = 156 cal. = 1 mile
Pilates	15 min. = 156 cal. = 1 mile
Raquetball (casual)	15 min. = 159 cal. = 1 mile
Stretching exercises	25 min. = 150 cal. = 1 mile
Weight lifting (also works for weight machines used moderately or gently)	30 min. = 156 cal. = 1 mile

Family Leisure

Playing piano	37 min. = 155 cal. = 1 mile
Jumping rope	10 min. = 152 cal. = 1 mile
Skating (moderate)	20 min. = 152 cal. = 1 mile
Swimming	
moderate	17 min. = 156 cal. = 1 mile
vigorous	10 min. = 148 cal. = 1 mile
Table tennis	25 min. = 150 cal. = 1 mile
Walk/run/play with kids	25 min. = 150 cal. = 1 mile